Run for Your Life

Run for Your Life

Mark Cucuzzella, M.D.

with Broughton Coburn

ALFRED A. KNOPF · NEW YORK · 2018

THIS IS A BORZOI BOOK
PUBLISHED BY ALFRED A. KNOPF

www.aaknopf.com

Knopf, Borzoi Books, and the colophon
are registered trademarks of Penguin Random House LLC.

Library of Congress Cataloging-in-Publication Data
Names: Cucuzzella, Mark, author.
Title: Run for your life / Mark Cucuzzella, M.D.
Description: First edition. | New York : Alfred A. Knopf, 2018. |
Includes bibliographical references and index.
Identifiers: LCCN 2017061533 (print) | LCCN 2017056684 (ebook) |
ISBN 9781101946305 (hardback) | ISBN 9781101946312 (ebook)
Subjects: LCSH: Running—Training. | Running—Physiological aspects. |
Running injuries—Prevention. | BISAC: HEALTH & FITNESS / Exercise. |
SELF-HELP / General. | SPORTS & RECREATION / Running & Jogging.
Classification: LCC GV1061.5 (print) | LCC GV1061.5 .C83 2018 (ebook) |
DDC 613.7/172—dc23
LC record available at https://lccn.loc.gov/2017061533

Jacket photograph by David Niblack/Imagebase.net
Jacket design by Carol Devine Carson

Manufactured in the United States of America

First Edition

Contents

Introduction

If we could give every individual the right amount of nourishment and exercise, not too little and not too much, we would have found the safest way to health.

—HIPPOCRATES

In college, a persistent dream captured many of my waking hours: to run with effortless, efficient grace.

But first, I had to figure out how to run without pain.

Getting to that point wasn't easy, nor did it happen quickly. I had to scrap my preconceptions and retool the way I stood, walked, and eventually ran. My roundabout path took me to medical school, to active-duty Air Force, to the University of Colorado, and to a rural West Virginia family medicine practice—via twenty-four Boston Marathons. Along the route, I picked up more tasks—as the U.S. Air Force's running coach, as a prof at the West Virginia University School of Medicine, as a race director, and as the owner-operator of an award-winning shoe store.

Eventually—and as something of a surprise—I reached a sustained high level of pain-free physical performance, accompanied by a remarkable sense of well-being. This sense of *wellness* is there for the learning and the taking. It requires little more than getting outside—moving, exercising, running, walking, and enjoying physical activity together.

The emphasis is on the *together* part. More important than any running achievements, I'm most proud of having initiated several community school and health programs, and founding one of the eastern seaboard's most popular fun runs. Throughout, my goal has been to help boost fitness and health for people of every age, and I've been encouraged by the testimonials from near-countless injured and sedentary folks who are now running, playing, and exerting with joy.

Distressingly, I've seen too many dedicated runners become former runners. And I've seen many nonrunners never begin. Too often in my medical practice I hear the phrase "I hate to run" or "I can't."

It doesn't need to be this way.

However odd it sounds, health care professionals are often complicit in unhealthy behavior and outcomes, by providing treatments that don't offer lasting solutions. When treating runners, we tend to ignore "prehab," the preventive solution: learn proper posture, strengthen the core muscles, settle into a good running pace, build endurance, understand mobility and efficiency of movement, and indulge a sense of contentment. Add to that restful sleep, good nutrition, sufficient recovery time, and even a sense of community, and you are solidly on the path to becoming stronger, to *preventing* injury, and to appreciating the magical gift of the human form. Simplicity of style begets efficiency of function.

The chapters of this book, and the exercises that conclude each of them, are designed to fit into your busy life. Nowadays, I can't imagine lining up for marathons and ultra distances without my secret weapon: the techniques that are summarized in this humble volume. By applying these principles, I now hold the world's longest active streak (thirty years) for consecutive years of running marathons in under 3 hours. At ages forty and forty-four, I won the Air Force Marathon outright in 2:31 and 2:38, and at age forty-four I ran the Boston Marathon in 2:34. I've also dabbled in ultra-marathons, including a first-place Masters finish in the competitive JFK 50 Mile run. My times are slowing a tad now that I've reached fifty (and my life becomes overfilled), but I anticipate many more years of running enjoyment. You can, too—whatever your performance goals.

You're invited to be my companion on this exhilarating path of self-discovery. For me, the discovery and learning continue—daily, at full throttle—as I devour emerging information on diet and diabetes, on our microbiome, on stress and stress relief, on the benefits of nature, and on much more. Simply put, we need to grab our kids and our old folks, get outside, and build movement, healthful food, and joy into our communities. It's not just about running. If you prefer to walk—or garden, or hike, or play golf—most of what you'll find here applies to you, too. My own path to these discoveries entailed endless trial and error. By reading this book, you'll leapfrog my struggle and experimentation to find an easier and faster way to a fit, healthy life. I'm grateful for the chance to share with you the secrets that I have learned.

AN ULTRA-MARATHON-LONG STORY

For me, running didn't happen in a straight line. I began to run at the age of thirteen, and often was the fastest in my age group. Modest successes generated enough positive reinforcement to keep me going, harder and faster. I competed through high school, and in the mid-1980s I raced for the University of Virginia.

But triumphs were well seasoned with pain, injuries, setbacks, surgeries, and lengthy rehab. I underwent my first knee surgery at age fifteen, and spent most of my high school years swimming laps at the YMCA instead of running. At one point, as a side effect of prescribed anti-inflammatories, I lost half my blood from an intestinal ulcer.

In 2000, arthritis in my big toes nearly ended my running career. That's when I attempted to qualify for the 2000 Olympic Trials. I had run the Military World Championship Marathon in 2:24, on a steamy hot day in Rome and with marginal training. Surely I could finish the racetrack-like Chicago Marathon in 2:22, the time needed to qualify. For six months I devoted all my spare time to training for the 1999 Chicago race.

Pain dictates your level of effort, and your joy. And in the six months preceding the Chicago Marathon, I hadn't strung together a single week of pain-free training. Plantar fasciitis nagged me with every step, even when walking.

I lined up, anyway, with the other competitors. I forced myself to maintain a pace of 5:20 for each of the first twenty miles, then began to slow. My final time of 2 hours and 24 minutes was respectable, but a couple of minutes shy of the qualifying time.

My next event was surgery—to relieve (some) of the pain in my foot. But the arthritis left my big toe joints inflexible and crooked. Along the way, I acquired an array of arch supports, orthotics, and oddly designed shoes, which I offered (with prayers for deliverance) to my altar of pain-free running. Doctors consistently told me to quit running and take up another activity. But I could find nothing as convenient, relaxing, and enjoyable—nothing that delivered the same feeling of overall freedom.

As a chronically injured runner, I realized that if I wanted to continue to run, something would have to change. While studying at UVA, I became the patient and guinea pig of Dr. Daniel Kulund, the track team's physician, and grew curious about his unorthodox methods for treating running injuries. He had me run in the college swimming pool—as is prescribed for horses in rehab—and his office featured a deep, hot tub–sized pool in which his athletes ran in place while tethered to the pool's side wall. Instead of the stiff orthotics often prescribed by trainers and doctors, he molded soft shoe inserts in a toaster oven. These tools and techniques, it turns out—and others that are outlined in this book—are now routinely used by competitive runners for training, and they have shown remarkable results in injury prevention.

My perpetual cycle of running, injury, treatment, and recovery inspired me to study medicine. And in my free time, I set out to retool how I ran. I dove into the rabbit hole of physiology and running science, and sought advice from the leading experts. A book called *Running and Being,* by the late Dr. George Sheehan, caught my attention. Sheehan stressed that understanding the mechanics of movement (and the root causes of running injuries, and their prevention) is the foundation for running pain-free, for life. Experts such as Michael Yessis, Arthur Lydiard, Dr. Ray McClanahan, Phil Maffetone, and Danny Dreyer stressed that runners could improve their performance and reduce injuries by focusing carefully and mindfully on their technique. Clinicians and researchers Dr. Casey Kerrigan, Dr. Daniel Lieberman, Dr. Irene Davis, and Jay Dicharry confirmed this.

Gradually, I began to see that a mere handful of easy and commonsense changes to my running form—summarized at the end of each chapter—might allow me to return to running, by softening the impact with the ground, and by utilizing spring and momentum to move more efficiently over the surface of the earth. Just like the greatest runners of the world.

Kenyan runners and Mexico's Tarahumara people were already long-distance-running legends. What made them such consistently good performers? The answer is that they had developed these techniques naturally and unconsciously—out of necessity, as part of daily life, and as a form of play. Aesthetically, too, their form was smooth, efficient, and beautiful, characterized by a springy stride, a quicker cadence, perfect body posture, and a relaxed smile. They landed with their weight near the middle of the foot, and closer to the point below the body's center of mass. They often ran barefoot or in sandals.

Modern shoes for these runners would be nothing more than awkward and bulky prosthetic devices interfering with their pureness of form. Yet many of these design features have been incorporated into modern running shoes—a subject we will return to in the chapter on feet.

This book, and my mission, is directed at making running safer and more fun, regardless of what shoes you wear. I may be the only physician in the country who also owns a shoe store! The American College of Sports Medicine recently published a position paper on footwear that confirms and underscores what our small store, Two Rivers Treads, has been doing for years.

I had to homeschool myself on all aspects of foot health, especially in terms of stance and gait and how the foot interacts with the ground. While I was studying the natural human running form, what amazed me most was that the traditional runners of Mexico and Kenya appeared to be completely *relaxed* and *happy*, in contrast to having the pained expressions of so many of my running friends. I believe that this is because they were engaged in doing precisely what humans were designed to do: run. In a traditional nomadic hunter-gatherer society, the stakes were high: an injury that curtailed the ability to run or walk long distances meant being left behind. To run was to live.

It wasn't only our premodern ancestors who ran in this natural manner. Kids still do, at least until encumbered by footwear. There is something here that we can learn—or relearn, rather—from our own children. In fact, everything I have to offer here will bring you closer to your experience of running as a child.

Medical school didn't provide many answers. Learning the names of the bones and muscles and tendons of the foot gave me little insight into how this remarkable biological machine actually *works*. Indeed, the foot—maybe the least understood of all moving body parts—is the orchestrator and foundation of all motion. What we *do* know is that it is superbly designed for its most important functions: absorbing shock, sending signals to the brain to maintain stability, and propelling the body forward.

Except in cases of structural deformities of the foot, modern shoes—inventions of the past thirty-plus years—haven't been able to improve upon the natural function of the over one-million-year-old human foot. Take a look at the chain of events that happen when you place your foot in a modern shoe: the heel is elevated, the toes are compressed, the arch of the foot is braced. All of this alters forces on the knees, hips, pelvis, and spine.

The arch, when confined within a non-anatomically shaped shoe, doesn't function in the manner it was designed for. And elevating the heel initiates a domino effect of compensations. Especially the great toe is dynamic and important. Overall, the resulting loss of foot stability is telegraphed up the kinetic chain of our bodies, tilting the pelvis, swaying the back, and shifting our center of mass forward—away from the critical area of the foot that is meant to bear weight. Our posture and gait are thrown out of whack. Picture an orderly stack of building blocks. Then elevate

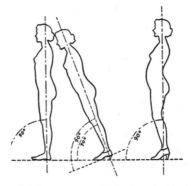

Introducing high heels causes the body to make adjustments
to posture that misalign the entire kinetic chain.

one edge of the bottom block. To restabilize the tottering stack, you'll likely need to make several adjustments, misaligning each piece slightly, from bottom to top.

Many runners have described the techniques outlined here as nothing less than life-changing. Admittedly, my wife, also a physician and researcher, remarked that "the plural of anecdote is not fact." She's right. So I launched studies of my own. In late 2007, Danny Dreyer, author of *ChiRunning,* and I surveyed twenty-five hundred runners who had adopted these techniques and presented the findings at scientific assemblies. We found that those who landed more on their midfoot while running ran more comfortably, suffered fewer injuries, and shared a feeling that they needed less effort to run. In 2012 I developed the Efficient Running Program for the U.S. Air Force—an interactive multimedia course designed to teach members of the military, as well as civilians, to be healthier and better runners.

There's more to healthy running and walking than footwear and biomechanics. Sports science legend Dr. Tim Noakes, a friend and colleague, stresses that what we are really training for is the maintenance of optimal health, and to live long and productive lives. That means that the best type of training is *the level of training that is sustainable.*

We now appreciate that the healthiest and often the fastest runners—those with consistently high performance and the fewest injuries—focus their training not on maximum speed but on *achieving maximum efficiency at the fully aerobic effort appropriate to each individual.* These athletes don't strive for *maximum* output. They tune their effort to their personal level of *sustained* output. This is the level of exertion at which our stores of fat are drawn upon as the primary, consistent fuel source—in preference to recently consumed and quickly metabolized sugars.

In the process of building the aerobic, fat-burning system to its highest potential, the runner becomes efficient in terms of both form and aerobic metabolism (conversion of sugars and fat, in the presence of oxygen, to energy). Over a long—but not exhausting—period of training, our bodies build millions of new capillary pathways for oxygen delivery. Paradoxically, in order to reliably increase performance, a runner actually needs to *slow down* and observe a modest speed limit, below the maximum level of effort.

As a physician, I have tried to ground my recommendations in science. Sports equipment design has been evolving for decades. Training regimens, and the level of play itself, have been changing and expanding. But sports medicine hasn't kept pace with these changes, and medical professionals have been slow to learn. Medical science and technology have advanced greatly, but running injuries are still treated with old-school remedies: enforced rest, ice packs, heavily cushioned shoes, orthotics, and stretching. *Despite all this care and intervention, more than half of all runners continue to be injured each year.* Pain relief is almost always temporary, and some medications, such as ibuprofen, actually inhibit healing and can prolong the recovery period.

Simply put, athletes and patients with running injuries receive too much *treatment* and not enough *attention* and *thought*. Medical schools and hospital residencies offer little guidance in the evaluation, prevention, and rehabilitation of overuse injuries. In med school, we learned how to treat *parts* of bodies (as if the body were a department store), not whole bodies. We were taught to treat the symptoms, not to address the underlying imbalances and weaknesses. True prevention means not allowing the condition to arise and develop in the first place. Take diabetes and heart disease. The best prevention is to eat a healthful diet, to avoid stress, and to go on a daily walk or run. And of course not to smoke.

The medical profession can begin by drawing nonphysicians—physiotherapists, podiatrists, coaches, media people, tech and engineering innovators, and runners themselves—into the discussion about why running injuries recur and persist. Their ideas, experience, and observations can help short-circuit the endless diagnostic duet that doctors and patients have been playing. This may not happen overnight. It normally takes ten years for an important medical discovery to become routine in a clinician's practice. Indeed, it was a decade before the modern protocol for the treatment of heart attacks was widely adopted by emergency departments.

What's needed is a new approach to running. Paradoxically, that approach involves *less* medical intervention for runners, not more.

As a family doc, I generally ask patients what physical activities they like do.

"Well, I can't run . . ." is a common response.

"Tell me a little more about that," I'll say.

Typically, they complain of suffering from a bad back, a bum knee, or pain in an ankle, then add, "My last doctor told me to do something safer." Or they simply say that running is too difficult and painful for them.

"Tell me some more about that," I'll press.

Inevitably, I discover that their lack of physical activity, unhealthy lifestyle, questionable diet, and prior physician's discouragement are largely to blame for their symptoms and the illness they are suffering.

This recurring clinical experience indicated to me that our community had the makings for a public health crisis, so I tried out some simple ways to address it. I taught courses in low-carb living, developed a series of community running events aimed at beginners, and hosted training clinics to prepare them for running safely. Then I opened a small retail run and walk center.

The more I examine patients and learn about how their bodies function and respond to stress, the more I realize that it's almost always possible to get into good running shape—safely. Humans were designed to run. Many more of us can run than believe we can.

Indeed, as a society, we *need* to run. The incidence of obesity has skyrocketed globally, and continues to climb. The Centers for Disease Control and Prevention estimate that more than one-third of U.S. adults and 20 percent of children and adolescents aged two to nineteen years are obese. That's 12.5 million kids. The American Heart Association recently reported that children today are ninety seconds slower on a one-mile run than their parents were at their age.

In our local running races and running clubs, I've observed that children don't *choose* to be obese and inactive. And they *love* to run. So I sparked a local initiative to build running trails at a dozen elementary schools, with daily activities scheduled on them. West Virginia recently mandated thirty minutes of activity per day for schoolchildren, and the trails facilitate this—without adding a burden on PE teachers or school resources. Cross-country running is now a sport at our area's middle schools, and has been wildly successful since the inaugural year, 2016, in Berkeley County.

These may be small, localized efforts, but our experience underscores that our community's public health challenge is shared nationwide. The obese and unfit are more likely to develop chronic diseases such as type 2 diabetes, heart disease, dementia, and certain types of cancer. Medical science has no pill or intervention that can reliably reverse the course of these chronic illnesses, but we can reverse much of them on our own: studies increasingly show that physical activity and improved nutrition yield the best results in terms of improving health, well-being, and longevity. As a physician, I can't help but prescribe *health* to my patients. In my mind, to *not* do so would violate the Hippocratic Oath.

Good nutrition is key. At the WVU School of Medicine, I'm co-directing a project, now in its fourth year, to not only teach students nutritional science, but to instruct them in cooking. In this book we'll show you how easy it is to eat healthfully: simply eat real food. Avoid sugar and processed ingredients, and load up on the natural nutrients available in plants, nuts, full-fat dairy, eggs, animals, and fish, if you choose. Modify a true Mediterranean- or Paleo-style or low-carb diet to your culture and tastes. We'll discuss this more in the chapters on diet and nutrition.

Humans can adapt. Almost twenty years ago, doctors advised me to quit running. Now I am running with a near-magical sense of well-being. It may sound like an extravagant claim, but running can be a comfortable, energizing, and fun activity for nearly anyone, at any age. In running, as in play, there doesn't need to be a measurable outcome. Simply put your foot down, maintain correct body position, and push and extend from the hips and glutes. Feel the spring. No stress, bending, or pain.

The adage *No pain, no gain* should be a thing of the past. *No pain, thank you*—this is the natural, healthy way. The goal doesn't have to do with running times. It's about health and well-being of the body and mind. Running, the activity that we humans are perhaps best adapted for, is a marvelous vehicle for this. It's a great place to start. And it's a great place to circle back to, again and again.

Run for Your Life is not a destination. It is a fun, relaxed journey. Try it and see where it takes you. Follow your body's feelings, and if they are positive, keep going! I'm confident that you'll discover that your legs and your body are a near-tireless vehicle—a parked hot rod that's ready to rev up, roll out, and speed you to a whole new level of health and satisfaction.

DRILLS

How can we become healthier, more efficient runners? The exercises presented at the end of the chapters that follow are designed to make you—as my colleague Jay Dicharry (author of *Anatomy for Runners*) has deftly outlined—

- *Smarter*—by using the illustrations to learn correct movement patterns;
- *Stronger*—by building endurance, strength, balance, and stability in key postural muscles;
- *Springier*—by gradually advancing and fine-tuning your workouts and daily movements, to leverage your body's natural springs.

The drills are easy to perform, and they generate little impact and stress, if done correctly and progressively. Specifically, in the drills and accompanying text, you will learn to:

- Breathe, sit, stand, and balance better throughout the day, and while running.
- Rebuild and maintain the essential range of motion of all your limbs.
- Bring strength and stability to your stance, and develop power in your hip extension.
- Set and maintain a consistent cadence, while feeling a springy "pop" off the ground.
- Run and move with comfort and joy, wanting more— even at the end of a workout.
- Eat and enjoy food that is tasty, nutritious, and inexpensive—and help reduce excess body fat.
- Learn ways to make your newly rediscovered health and vigor more accessible to others, and pay it forward to improve the health of your community.

The goal, during the running-oriented exercises, is to master the movements and maintain proper form—and then build more speed and power into that form. *Less,* done correctly, is better than *more,* done incorrectly. As your strength and neuromuscular sense grow, you'll find that the natural "springs" in your legs and body become stronger and smarter. Eventually, a properly performed drill *becomes* your running form.

The drills that you select can be performed as infrequently as twice a week, requiring no more than fifteen minutes each time. They are best done on days when you are not fatigued, and after you have warmed up. Begin by picking some exercises that look easy, and graduate to more challenging ones that play to your weaknesses—until they become your strengths.

Consider this book a user-friendly owner's manual to the body, dedicated to the safe operation and maintenance of the gift we have been given. Thankfully, you don't have to follow a tight regimen—but you do need to stick with it. If you suffer from a shortage of time, then take any opportunity to skip, jump, spring, and balance during your daily life. The drills and "exercise snacks" in the pages that follow can be surprisingly fun and energizing, if done with a little patience and good form. You are training, after all, for the rest of your hopefully long and healthy life.

PART I

Before the Starting Line

CHAPTER 1

Our Bodies Are Older Than We Think

Nothing in biology makes sense except in the light of evolution.
—THEODOSIUS DOBZHANSKY

MYTH: *Life spans have increased compared with decades ago.*

FACT: *When chronic disease and declining public health are factored in, modern life spans aren't much longer than they used to be. By some measures, average functional life spans in the United States have started to decline.*

Whether your goal is athletic dominance or simply to arrive at a healthy old age, we all share the goal of making the best of our lives while on the planet, in the healthiest and most productive way that we can.

Let's start by inspecting the miraculous equipment we inherited, to better understand what it is that our bodies were designed to do.

RUNNING IS ONLY HUMAN

Throughout human history—for almost 2 million years as hunter-gatherers, followed by 12,000 years as pastoralists and farmers—our ability to run, to walk, and to be physically active has been essential to life. By virtue of our existence—indeed, as evidenced by our domination of the planet—humans are succeeding. So far, at least.

Our prehuman, primate ancestors were slower and weaker than many of the large animals that they eventually would learn to prey upon. Masters of agility, their bodies and limbs were adapted mainly for living in trees, where they could find forage and fruit, and were safe from nonclimbing predators that lived on the forest floor.

So how did they come to dominate these other species, prey upon them, and even drive some of them to extinction? And later, what enabled modern humans, *Homo sapiens,* to win the evolution race with earlier species of our genus? Was it brains over brawn, or the other way around? Or did our brawn and brains coevolve?

By nearly every metric of human strength and performance, early hominids (and even one extinct line, the Neanderthals) were superior to *Homo sapiens.* We made an incremental yet critical adaptation by gradually becoming able to walk and run long distances.

Scientists generally believe that the ability to walk and run on two feet was a game changer. With the rudimentary tools available to early humans, it would have been difficult and dangerous to bring down an antelope. Yet there's evidence that humans were

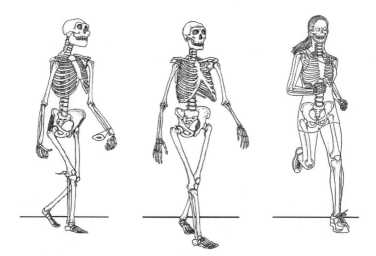

The ability to walk and run long distances was a game changer for our ancestors.

killing and eating large prey for some time *before* spears and other weapons were developed.

One compelling theory proposes that early humans' ability to walk (and occasionally run) long distances in hot climates allowed them to track large, fast prey until the animals dropped of heat exhaustion and dehydration, unable to run or to fight. Doing so at a walking pace wouldn't have been sufficient. Early humans sprinted when escaping a predator or other imminent dangers. But when tracking game, according to the "persistence hunting" theory, they would have needed to travel only fast enough to keep their prey moving and not resting. (Most large animals shed heat by panting, yet they are unable to pant while running.)

Our ability to travel long distances in an energy-efficient manner helped us with more than hunting. It also allowed us to relocate more readily to a new water source, for instance, or travel to a more bountiful area. Essentially, we could walk away from perils such as famine and drought, sometimes to distant locations, aided by an ability to efficiently store and utilize the calories we consumed.

WE GOT THE RIGHT GEAR

Dr. Dan Lieberman and colleagues have identified evolutionary adaptations in our anatomy and physiology that enhance our ability to walk and run long distances. Mainly, we benefited from the following features, which you may even begin to notice as you pay attention to your running:

- Springy *tendons and muscles in the legs* that work in efficient harmony. As the springlike, fibrous tendons stretch, they load up with potential energy. The muscles contribute to stability at the same time that the tendons spring us forward.
- Extra-large *gluteus maximus*, or butt muscles, that make for strong and stable hips and trunk.
- An *upright posture*, *exceptional balance*, and a *stable head and neck*. Notice that these features enable us, while running on two feet, to remain simultaneously aware of our surroundings and focused on a distant object. Some

believe that our well-developed vestibular system (the region of the inner ear that controls balance) may have contributed substantially to our survival success.

- *Sweat glands*, which humans have an abundance of. Sweating provides effective evaporative cooling, or thermoregulation. We adapt to heat by perspiring more as the temperature and our activity levels rise. Our absence of fur, minimal body hair, and high surface-area-to-body-weight ratio mean that more skin is exposed to the air's cooling effect. Also, uniquely, our breathing pattern is uncoupled from our stride, so we can unload body heat through our lungs during respiration, which four-legged mammals cannot.

- The *capacity to digest, store, and utilize fat* as an efficient source of fuel. Fat contains twice the calories per gram as sugar. That fat is metabolized with seven to ten times greater efficiency than sugar, too. (We'll explore this valuable fuel source in the chapters on endurance and nutrition.)

- *Feet that are uniquely adapted to walking and running, with their springlike arches and short toes.* Each foot is an orchestra of 26 bones, 33 joints, 107 ligaments, and 19 muscles and tendons, providing cushioning, spring, and control in three planes simultaneously. Chapter 4 is devoted to this remarkable appendage.

SLOW, BUT SMART

Despite all of our evolutionary adaptations, humans would appear to be physiologically flawed. Raising our young to adulthood requires (nonproductive) years of nurturing and training, and our top speed is slow when compared to similar-sized wild animals.

Natural selection entails trade-offs and compromise. Humans have developed great endurance, but we aren't very fast. (The fastest land animal, the cheetah, is specialized for catching prey with speed but has little endurance.) And the human ability to efficiently store fat is useful for surviving famines, yet comes with

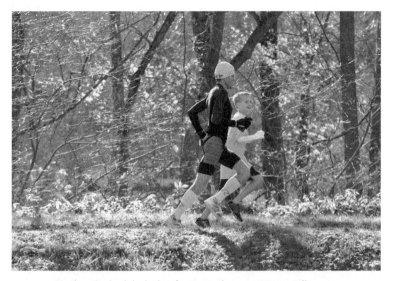

Testing the body's design features: the 2015 JFK 50 Mile race.
It requires good posture, springy legs, stability from the glutes,
efficient energy use, and a mix of walking and running.

a high risk of obesity. Even brain size offers a trade-off: the large human brain is a hungry organ, consuming about a quarter of the body's resting energy demand—diverting calories that might be more productively dedicated to strength and speed.

Nonetheless, our brains have served us well. Our evolving brains led to the harnessing of fire, and the cooking, grinding, and mashing of foods with tools. Softening tough plant and animal fibers sped up the process of chewing and digestion, so greater quantities of protein and fat can be metabolized by the body. (Cooked foods yield more than twice the usable nutrition of raw foods: cellulose and the proteins of muscle fiber denature at high temperatures, making them softer and easier for the body to digest.)

The nutritional boost from consuming higher-quality food supported the development of *more* brain power. As humans grew smarter, their socialization, hunting skills, and tool-making abilities improved. Meanwhile, the control of fire helped with more than cooking: the deterrent effect of fire on wild animals allowed humans to sleep longer without fear of predators. Deeper REM sleep further aided brain function and growth.

Along the way, humans became fat-storing and fat-burning

machines. Fats and proteins offer the critical building blocks for brain and muscle, and fat is more energy- and essential nutrient–dense than carbohydrates. The Inuit, for example, remained healthy without consuming *any* carbohydrates. Humans cannot survive without fat.

Early humans also developed an ability to store (energy-poor) carbohydrates by efficiently *converting* them to (energy-rich) fat, with the help of insulin. In times of plenty we could accumulate fat, then metabolize it in times of need—drawing upon it over periods without food, if necessary, before needing to "refuel."

NURTURE OR NATURE?

Individual performance varies, and this variation can be partly explained by genes. But lifestyle, diet, and behavior matter, too. A journalist named Adharanand Finn observed the strenuous, physically active lives of rural Kenyan children, many of whom chase goats and livestock at home, then run long distances to and from school. These children have little access to television or computers, and virtually all of them are barefoot. One Kenyan tribe in particular has consistently produced running champions—the Kalenjin. Their steely determination and active rural lifestyle appear to have converged to make them the fastest endurance runners in the world.

Similarly, the Tarahumara of Mexico are famous for covering extraordinary distances wearing sandals made of old tires and rope. When Tarahumara legend Arnulfo Quimare spoke at the 2016 Boston Marathon, a runner in the audience asked about his "training" regimen. Through a translator (who had to pause to find the suitable word), Arnulfo replied that his "training" consisted mostly of *walking* from village to village.

When it comes to running, there's no evidence that the Tarahumara or the Kenyans are genetically superior to anyone else. Harvard evolutionary biologist Daniel Lieberman points out that people in these groups are prone, like all of us, to habits that can lead to illness and poor running technique, especially when they adopt Western diets and modern running shoes.

COMPETING EVOLUTIONARY INTENTIONS

We *evolved* to run, to walk, and to remain active. At the same time, we were *born* to conserve energy whenever possible—to rest and relax. In the calorie-shy world of our ancestors, the ability to reduce caloric expenditure, and to *store* that energy through periods of no food, conferred survival advantages. For modern humans, however, this genetic tendency to pack away calories has created something of an evolutionary dilemma. Researcher James H. O'Keefe and his colleagues describe a "millennia-old connection—the balance between energy expenditure, calorie ingestion, and appropriate hormonal responses." In other words, the connection between our inner nature and the environment we live in has largely been severed. "Until a century or so ago," O'Keefe says, "never before in history have humans been routinely exposed to high caloric, highly processed foods in excess of the calories needed to function." (This may have been true for most, but not all. Dr. Michael Eades often speaks of the mummified evidence and artistic renditions of the farinaceous Egyptian culture. A high body weight may have been a sign of wealth and status, though it appears that a far smaller percentage of people were overweight in earlier times.)

We're beginning to see that this inborn proclivity to take the path of least resistance and eat as much as we desire plays a major role in the health woes and rising health care costs beleaguering modern people. Obesity and high-sugar diets create fertile ground for a variety of modern diseases, especially type 2 diabetes. We'll address this in the chapters on nutrition and diet.

Therein lies the inspiration for this book: the hope that we can become better, more functional, healthier humans—and restore and nurture our connection to who we are and to how we were meant to live. This doesn't mean finding a place of stasis and comfort. It demands that we actively *resist* the inborn desire to remain on the couch and eat whatever is within reach.

We're living in a unique time in human history, one in which we have a choice of lifestyles. Our bodies didn't evolve to sit all day at a desk, though many of us do. Nor, admittedly, did we evolve to be ultra-marathon-running machines, though I have occasionally aspired to be such, and have enjoyed the adventure. Our goal should be to find a place in between, and to adopt a lifestyle that matches what our bodies were designed for. Homeostasis with hormesis as the path to excellence.

NEW OLD ROUTINES

The daily routines we have fallen into over the past several generations have perpetuated a number of habits that are harmful to our health. Not only have our diets, sleep patterns, and anxiety levels changed, but the ways we move our bodies (or don't move them) have drifted from the natural, ergonomically efficient patterns of our ancestors. One example is *sitting*, which I discuss in chapter 3, on posture and walking. If we sit in a slumped position—head and shoulders forward, hips flexed, and glutes overstretched—we develop a muscle memory that disrupts our standing posture. We become misaligned, and all of our movements suffer.

Technological aids and interventions don't help. Drugs, orthotics, gimmicks, supplements, and fads that promise to compensate for our declining mobility and health mainly serve to accelerate our bodies' physiological drift. These expensive "fixes" seldom correct the underlying problems, which often originate in poor posture, incorrect movement, and unhealthy behavior. Many of the modern medical interventions, too, merely accommodate our ancient human bodies to a very different modern world. We end up with growing instances of what Dr. Lieberman has termed "mismatch diseases," afflictions resulting from behavior, movement patterns, and diet that don't match the physiology (and psychology) of the bodies and minds we inherited from our ancestors.

QUALITY OF LIFE: MORE IMPORTANT THAN QUANTITY

Despite all this medical attention, the disability-adjusted life expectancy (DALE) and the health-adjusted life expectancy (HALE) for Americans is only seventy years, which doesn't even figure into the global top twenty. And if you discount only two developments of the last century—the significant reduction in infant mortality, and the singular lifesaving qualities of antibiotics—life spans today aren't all that much longer than they were generations ago.

By some measures, average *functional* life spans in the United States have started to decline. This refers to the length of one's healthy, active life, in contrast to the total number of years that one has been alive. In light of this, Orville Rogers, a one-hundred-year-old Masters record holder in the 200-meter run, quipped that our goal should be to "live long and die short."

How do we do that? Researcher James O'Keefe points out that the daily physical activity pattern of hunter-gatherers forms an ideal template from which to design a modern exercise regimen—one that works to realign our daily movement with the archetype encoded within our genome. Indeed, the drills at the end of each chapter have premodern counterparts. For instance, endurance training (long, slow runs) was essential for persistence hunting; interval training (jogging punctuated with short sprints) corresponds to fighting and fleeing; strength training (such as lifting weights) replicates house building or handling large game; and mobility training (moving the body through its full range of motion) reproduces a variety of movements needed for survival. *Rest and recovery* is included front and center in this template: hunter-gatherers spent plenty of time relaxing, too.

I'm convinced that to avoid the tantalizing perils of the convenient modern age, we need to reclaim a bit of our evolutionary past—by eating simple, natural foods, and by regularly putting our bodies through a wide range of movements. Throughout, hopefully, we'll also experience a sense of *enjoyment* and *play*. (In recent generations, this has been re-created in the context of sports.)

Fortunately, even low to moderate levels of exercise, sports, or exertion at your job can improve your health. This simple message isn't always self-evident in a society that assumes more is better and faster is best. As a doctor attempting to reintroduce the concepts of simplicity, consistency, and modest effort, I sometimes feel "old school," swimming against a tide of fads, assumptions, quick fixes, hacks, New Age remedies, and popular theories.

You're about to learn more about the miracle of human mechanics and enjoy the art, the mechanics, and the plain old addictive pleasure of walking and running, which is ingrained in our DNA.

Let's get started.

DRILLS

The preliminary drills in this chapter involve balance, which requires the integration of our eyes, inner ears, and receptors in our feet and throughout the body. Balance is the foundation—the prerequisite, really—for the other exercises and activities described in this book. And good balance is the basis of healthy running's single most important attribute: relaxation.

Once you have mastered the drills below, you can elevate the challenge and add a bit of fun by closing your eyes, or by standing on a cushion or folded yoga mat.

One-legged balance

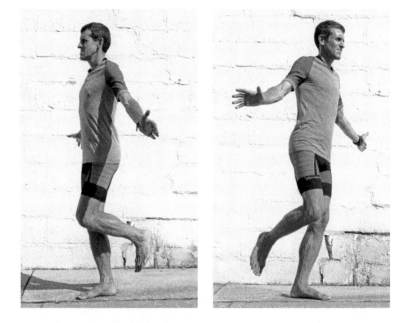

Start barefoot on a firm surface. Keep a chair or a wall within reach.

Lift your knee and lower leg slightly. Then slowly lower and extend your thigh behind you, and extend it at the hip. Hold this position first with eyes open, then closed. Change up your position by placing your hands on your hips, by stretching your arms to the side, and by swinging them up and down (as if making "snow angels" in the air), with your thumbs pointed to the rear. Switch feet. Repeat this as often as you can during the day.

Leg swings

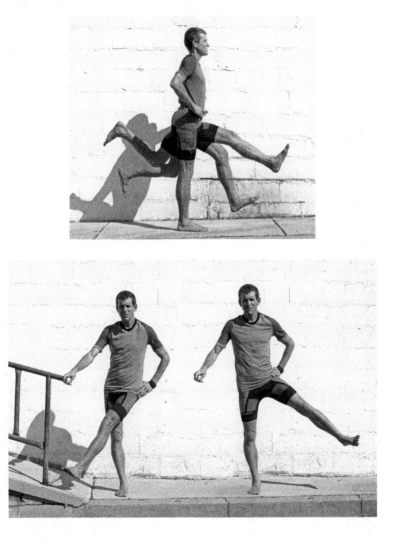

Stand on your right leg and raise the left leg a few inches off the floor. With arms at your sides, swing your left leg forward and back, then from side to side. Repeat with the other leg. Try not to allow your swinging foot to touch the ground.

One-legged squat

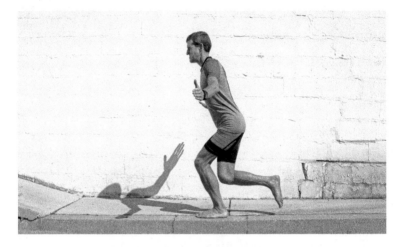

Plant your feet hip-width apart. Lift your right foot and extend it back just a bit. Now push your hips back and down into a partial, one-legged squat position. Your right knee is bent, chest upright, eyes forward, as your butt aims for an imaginary stool behind you. Use your glutes (butt muscles) to return to the starting position. Repeat with the other foot.

Golfer's pickup (or single-leg dead lift)

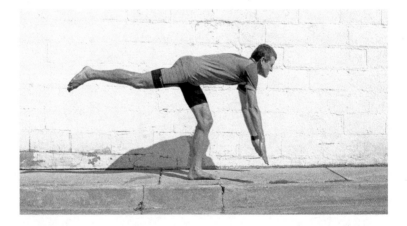

As you hinge forward, maintain a straight line from your head to your outstretched foot. Keep your hips parallel to the floor, and maintain the natural lumbar curve of your back.

For repeated lifting from the floor of light objects (only!), the safest method is *not* to bend the knees and to keep the back erect. The "golfer's pickup" is easier on the joints. As one leg rises behind (for counterbalance), the torso tilts forward over the stance leg, forming a fulcrum. No spine or knee bending occurs.

Simply balance on your left foot and hinge forward at the hips, while you reach toward the ground with your right hand as if to pick up a golf ball. Your knee and your back are straight but relaxed throughout. Tighten the buttocks as you return to the starting position.

Explore your feet

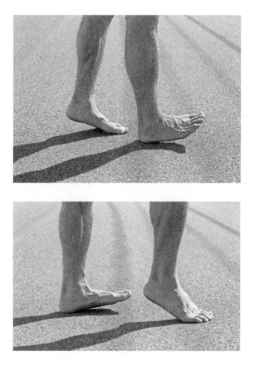

Our feet have two hundred thousand sensory receptors that are constantly, and unconsciously, apprising us of our position so that we can make microadjustments to our balance. With your shoes off, in the house or in the office, spend a bit of time each day walking on your heels, then on the balls of your feet, then on the outside edges of the feet, then on the inside edges.

Single-leg run (for the more advanced)

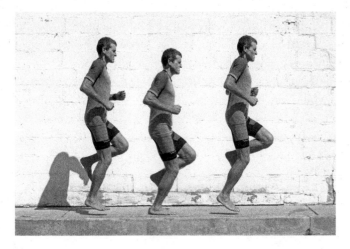

I do this several times a week at the end of a run, preferably on a soft (but not unstable) surface such as a grassy field. Balance on one leg, engage the muscles of your core, and hop with a running motion on one leg for five to ten hops. Switch to the other leg. Start with 10–20 meters, and work your way up to 50–100 meters. This requires active concentration on balance, and focusing on the foot and lower leg as a spring.

CHAPTER 2

Stand Up and Breathe

Eighty percent of young people have back pain. The other 20 percent have no computer.

—UNKNOWN

MYTH: *Strength is the foundation of performance.*

FACT: *It all begins with posture.*

I live in West Virginia, but when I run in Central Park, I pause at the "Imagine" mosaic that memorializes John Lennon, and I imagine peace in the world. I also imagine a world in which we are more at peace with our own bodies. It's a world where there is no back pain, and no metabolic or degenerative illnesses.

That world exists today—for societies in which people avoid prolonged *sitting*. If you are in your early fifties or older, you may even remember that time—a pre-video-game childhood of summers when the only occasion you sat was at the table for dinner (and maybe on the floor for a board game or an episode of your favorite TV show).

Now we suffer through chronic back pain, poor posture, and incomplete breathing, much of it caused by too much sitting. The good news is that there are simple remedies for these, and they *add* time to your day, not take it away. All it requires is correcting your posture, spending more time on your feet, finding a bit of comfortable space on the floor, and working on "spine hygiene."

As John Lennon sings, *It's easy if you try*.

HOW SITTING IS KILLING US

Parking ourselves in chairs for extended periods results in a chronic shortening of the hip flexors, the muscles in front that connect the pelvis and lower spine to our legs. Sitting also overstretches and weakens the muscles in back, the glutes—the substantial butt muscles that support much of our movement. When we stand up after hours of being chair-bound, our pelvis and spine don't immediately return to their balanced, "neutral" position. Our posture remains stooped (sometimes imperceptibly) and our full range of motion is impaired.

This new "default" posture sets off a series of other postural compensations. Without fully realizing it, we end up walking around just slightly "wonky," with shoulders rolled forward, upper back rounded, and head carried in front of our center of

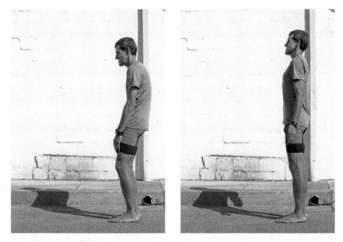

At left, head and shoulders are slumped forward in "texting position."
The spine is displaced from its natural, tall, straight architecture. Texting or desktop posture is hard on the joints and requires static muscle strength to maintain. On the right: straight, strong, and stable posture.

gravity—as shown in the figure on page 18. For every inch that your head is positioned forward, five to seven pounds of stress are added to the lower cervical spine. As we will learn in the chapter on feet, modern shoes (and elevated heels in particular) exacerbate this dysfunctional posture.

We simply spend too much time out of balance. When our posture is not tall, balanced, and relaxed, our efficiency of movement is reduced to the point that even standing becomes uncomfortable. This mild discomfort reinforces the desire to sit. As sitting becomes the easy, less painful option, it becomes habitual, and creates a *sedentary feedback loop*. As athlete and massage therapist Laura Bergman says, "How you stand is how you land." Cycling—though unquestionably a healthful activity—doesn't help with this, due to the cyclist's bent-over, sitting position.

Kids who are confined to school desks for hours (typically followed by more hours on couches at home) quietly begin to suffer a shortening of the deep hip flexors—the psoas and iliacus muscles. Distressingly, the resulting bent-over posture and inefficient movement patterns are imprinted and passed on to adulthood.

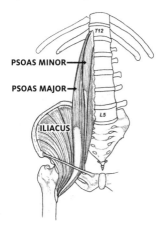

The iliacus and psoas are dominant hip flexors.
These major muscles shorten with prolonged sitting.

Physical therapist Kelly Starrett noticed that pre-kindergarten children run naturally, with minimal exertion—sprinting, powering hard, running on the balls of their feet, "like miniature Kenyan marathon runners." He also saw, as I have seen in my clinic, that by first grade half the kids start heel striking. And by second grade, most children's running and movement patterns have become dysfunctional. In this case, practice doesn't make perfect. It makes dysfunctionality permanent.

SITTING SENDS A SIGNAL: STORE UP THE CALORIES

In addition to the structural changes caused by sitting, the mere act of sitting down sends metabolic signals to *store energy*. As we'll explore later, sitting and inactivity trigger a dramatic reduction of the enzyme that is essential for the metabolism of triglycerides in muscle mitochondria. Those triglycerides are then converted into fatty acids that accumulate in the liver and in adipose tissues (belly fat), elevating the risk of metabolic diseases. Studies show that prolonged sitting decreases the diameter of arteries, as well, and increases blood pressure and the risk of heart disease, type 2 diabetes, cancer, and early death.

The bigger picture is even scarier. A recent meta-analysis, extracted from multiple studies and pooled data, showed that *even rigorous daily exercise doesn't mitigate the negative health effects of sitting,* even for those who exercise regularly and are physically active (including marathon runners). This "active couch potato syndrome" came as a surprise to me because, like many of us, I assumed that a daily thirty-minute run or other activity (as recommended in the *Physical Activity Guidelines for Americans*) would surely undo the harmful effects of a day of prolonged sitting.

As part of my Air Force flight doctor training, I spent one of the most physically challenging (and body-damaging) days of my life when I was subjected to repeated spins in a human centrifuge. I was taken up to six Gs (six times the force of gravity), then to nine Gs. I survived the test protocol, but the soreness I felt, which lasted several days, made a marathon seem like a Sunday stroll. Our bodies are simply not adapted to this kind of stress.

Joan Vernikos, former director of NASA's Life Sciences Division and author of *Sitting Kills, Moving Heals,* has studied the effects of G forces and gravity—and also weightlessness—on the body. She learned that prolonged zero gravity (no G forces) is *harder* on the body than those excessive G forces. Even relatively short periods in a weightless environment accelerate aging and reduce bone mass and bone mineral density, and this elevates the risk of fracture.

One G and hops of two and three Gs are fine! Gravity is magic, and fun. The most exciting, thrilling activities of earthbound folks involve gravity—managing it, leveraging it, playing with it, trying to defy it. Children understand this innately. Adults sometimes overlook this magic, and they lumpishly resign themselves to gravity's downward pull. Without even trying, simply by relaxing for hours in chairs, most of us are contributing to a medical study topic that I call "zero-G sedentary physiology." The science behind this is clear: prolonged sitting is harmful. We simply weren't designed to sit all day. Prolonged bed rest, too—our closest everyday proxy for zero G—should be banned from health care in almost every instance in which the patient can sit, stand, or walk.

"Gravity plays a big role in our physiological function, and in the aging process," Dr. Vernikos says. "We are not designed to exist in quasi-microgravity. We were designed to squat. We were designed to kneel. Sitting is okay, but it is *uninterrupted* sitting that's bad for us. And it's not *how many* hours of sitting that's bad for you; it's *how often you interrupt* that sitting that is *good* for you!"

DON'T TAKE THIS GOOD NEWS SITTING DOWN

Fortunately, the negative effects of sitting are reversible, and the solution is surprisingly easy: mix it up. If you have a cubicle job, merely *standing up* from a seated position (at least once every twenty minutes) actively helps your body to burn fat. Create a "dynamic" workstation that allows (and perhaps demands) you to change positions throughout the day. Or, if you're constantly on your feet—working in retail, for instance—take brief sitting breaks.

In a brilliant move, Kelly Starrett, who compared preschool and primary school kids, convinced his children's school to use stand-up desks—and they love them! A school in our town is using these now, too.

Standing all day in a static position isn't good, either. If you try a standing or treadmill desk—I highly recommend them—then be sure to take *some* time to sit and relax. And you can break up a standing position by alternately elevating a leg on a stool, chair, or windowsill, and slowly stretching the hip flexors. Take advantage of any brief gaps (while cogitating, for instance, or talking on the phone) to squat or to kneel. Mix it up, too. Walk around. If appropriate, lie prone to type or to read, or to play a game.

AVOID SITTING BACK

Not surprisingly, we suffer from a near epidemic of lower back pain. Lumbar pain is one of the leading causes of disability in the military and the civilian population, and it accounts for uncountable days of lost productivity. Treatment for back pain is an $80-billion-a-year industry, despite a growing medical consensus that most modern interventions, from injections to surgeries, have little or no value, and often cause harm.

We need to *treat the position, not the condition.* Standing up, paying attention to posture, stretching, squatting, and walking are the best ways to maintain good "spine hygiene." For those who have suffered a back injury or undergone back surgery, the best way to rehabilitate, generally, is to rebuild strength: to bend and twist and subject the spine to natural stresses and loads. Modern medicine doesn't offer spine transplants.

RELEARNING TO BREATHE

Good posture can't occur without proper abdominal (belly) breathing, because an engaged diaphragm is the key to stabilizing the core. When you allow the lower belly to fill as you inhale, your powerful diaphragm contracts and you fill the lower areas of the lungs, where maximum oxygen exchange occurs. As your abdomen fills, your upright core stiffens like a pressurized soda can. Notice those around you. Most are breathing from the upper chest, not from the diaphragm and abdomen.

Try breathing through your nose. This forces the diaphragm to work, and allows your carbon dioxide level to rise naturally, which assists in offloading oxygen to the tissues. Sufficient levels of car-

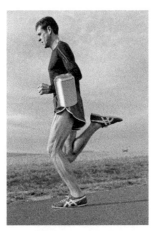

As you inhale and fill your lower abdomen with air,
your torso stiffens like a pressurized soda can,
stabilizing your core and allowing better oxygenation.

bon dioxide allow the body to utilize oxygen, so we need to make sure that we have enough CO_2 in our blood. Blowing off excessive CO_2 causes oxygen to bind to the hemoglobin rather than be released to the muscles and other tissues, where it should go. This is why you feel lightheaded when you overbreathe: not enough oxygen is offloading and reaching the brain, because you're expelling too much CO_2.

Slow, mindful breathing also triggers a soothing parasympathetic response, bringing sustained calm—and performance, too. In most athletic endeavors (outside of those involving only a second or two of explosive power), we perform better when we relax the body. Even in a sprint, Olympian Usain Bolt is relaxed as he accelerates. Michael Jordan's routine, prior to nailing almost every free throw (regardless of what the opposing fans were yelling at him), relied upon taking deep, slow breaths.

In my medical practice, I commonly see patients with respiratory problems that originate in poor breathing habits. Doctors often treat these patients symptomatically with inhalers, which often stimulate overbreathing. We should be teaching the skill of mindful, diaphragmatic breathing, in combination with an erect, relaxed, balanced posture.

DRILLS

1. Try these antidotes to the epidemic of sitting

There are several habits that you can introduce to your workday that will enhance your productivity, health, and enjoyment. Most important, stand or walk for at least half the day, and avoid sitting for more than twenty minutes at a stretch. If you have to work at a job that involves sitting for long periods, here are a few ways to keep from succumbing to the "sedentary feedback loop":

- *Work at a standing desk.* Several years ago, I stacked shoeboxes on my desk at work as a way to elevate my laptop. Now, West Virginia University has installed several stand-up stations, and the U.S. Air Force is embracing them. Be sure to move around, elevate a leg, and stretch whenever you can as you work.
- *Test run a treadmill desk.* You might have a friend or colleague who has one. Give it a try, for at least a half hour, at a variety of moderate speeds between 1 and 2.4 miles per hour. Remember to maintain proper, erect posture and breathe slowly and deeply. There's a good chance you'll feel more productive.
- *Walk or ride an elliptical bicycle to work.* An elliptical bike is essentially an indoor elliptical trainer mounted on an extended traditional bicycle frame. Some elite runners use them to cross-train, and for nonimpact cardio workouts. This isn't always realistic, but with a bit of creativity it can fit into at least part of a daily routine—for instance by driving part of the way to work, and walking or cycling or elliptical biking the rest.
- *Take standing or walking breaks.* Stand up for at least two out of every thirty minutes. If possible (while talking on the phone, for instance), walk outside, squat a few times, do some light stretching, dictate email replies on your phone, or have a walking meeting. Movement boosts cognitive processes. As a

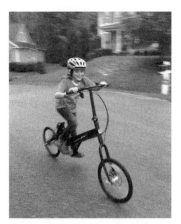

My ten-year-old daughter, Lily, takes a spin
on an elliptical bike. Look, Ma—no seat!

reminder, try setting a half-hour alarm on your phone
each time you sit down, or use an app like Time Out
(Mac) or Workrave (Windows).

- *Stand up at meetings.* If you're worried about what your
colleagues think, tell them you have a bad back! Better
yet, hold walking meetings.

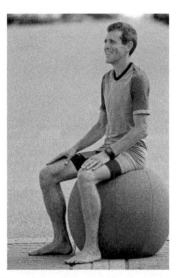

The back does not need "support" when sitting correctly.
Sitting erect will alleviate back pain and promote overall health.

- *Sit more actively.* Slumping passively in a chair isn't the only way to sit. Sit tall, with head erect, balanced directly over your "sitz" bones. Better yet, try sitting on a yoga ball or stool instead of a chair, which activates several sets of muscles—the ones needed to make small postural adjustments. (Venn Design makes one upholstered brand of this.) For car and airplane seats, I use a product called Backjoy, which better positions the pelvis and lower spine.)
- *Sit on the floor* whenever you can, and mix up the positions. This mobilizes your joints, muscles, and fascia, from toes to torso, and recruits important stabilizing muscles. The simple acts of sitting and arising are great for your body as well.

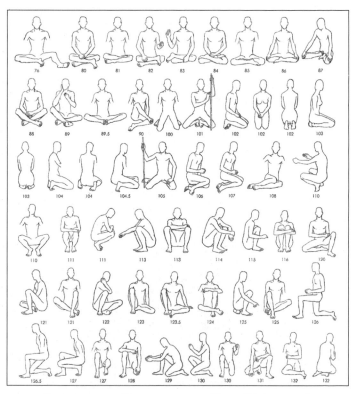

Here are some of the numerous positions—"sitting yoga,"
if you will—for sitting on the floor. (Kids naturally use many of these.)

2. Reset your standing posture

This entails more relaxation and alignment than it does effort. Throughout, inhale and exhale slowly and deeply with the diaphragm.

- Stand against a wall. Visualize good posture as a straight line that runs through your shoulder, hip, and ankle.
- Position your feet under your hips, thigh-width apart. Ideally, they should point forward, but don't force this—your natural position may be slightly splayed. Imprint this position in your memory. Through practice and repetition, you will create a new "normal." This may appear or feel stiff at first, because it's not how most people tend to stand. (When your feet point forward, as we'll see later, the arch of your foot is stable, which helps engage the powerful hip and glute muscles.)
- Balance on each foot's "tripod": the inner and outer edges of the feet (at the ball), and the heel. Place your

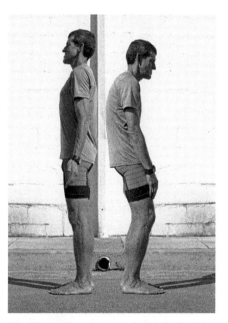

Begin by "standing tall" against a wall. Head, shoulders, buttocks, and heels should touch the wall, with space to slide your hand behind the small of your back. Then replicate that position without the wall.

feet hip-width apart, facing forward. Lock your knees. Now unlock them. Do you feel the difference? Flexible, unlocked knees give you stability. Let them relax into the most stable position.

- Now lengthen the back of your neck and *make yourself tall,* as if pulling yourself upward from the crown of your head. Your chin will naturally drop down.
- Reach up, as if for a cookie jar on a high shelf, and feel your spine lengthen (especially in the rib cage area). Maintain that elongated spine, and lower your arms.
- With your arms at your sides, roll your shoulders forward, then up, then back, and let your shoulder blades slide down your rib cage. Imagine that you are setting your shoulder blades the way an Old West outlaw returns his guns to his holsters. Boom! Stable shoulders.

Your posture should now be connected and straight: Hips over ankles. Shoulders over hips. Ears over shoulders. You should feel most of your weight on your heels. Picture yourself as *squarely balanced beneath your head.* If in doubt, have someone take a photo of you from the side, and see if the dots connect in a straight line— ears, shoulders, hips, ankles.

Your spine is now elongated and your diaphragm engaged. There's a simple test to confirm this: have someone stand behind you and push straight downward on your shoulders. If you collapse backward, tilt your torso slightly forward *from the hips,* and recheck. Find your stable column.

3. Reset your breathing

The short, diaphragmatic breathing drill on the videos page of the book's website (runforyourlifebook.com) will align and lengthen your spine, activate your diaphragm, enhance oxygenation of your tissues, and release buckets of parasympathetic hormones (the good stuff that relaxes you). It's a great way to bracket the start and end of your day.

- Slowly, lie down flat on your back. As in the photo on page 29, slide your feet toward your butt until your legs

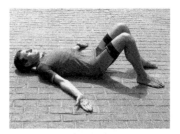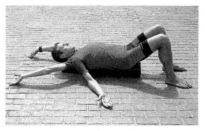

Lengthen your spine, tuck your shoulder blades, and breathe through the belly. Or, you can lie on a long foam roller and move your arms as if making a snow angel while deep breathing.

are bent at 90 degrees. Now try to lengthen your spine by imagining gentle traction pulling from the top of your head, stretching you into a fully lengthened position.

- Place your palms out and arms straight, as if making a snow angel, and tuck your shoulder blades under you.
- As a visual reference, place your phone or other small object on your belly button. It will rise and fall as you breathe in and out.
- Breathe all the way out, as if blowing up a balloon. Gently purse your lips to add a bit of controlled resistance, while centering your focus. To a slow count (*one thousand, two thousand, three thousand . . .*), now inhale into the abdomen through your nose.
- Pause at the top of the breath—then inhale just a bit more. This will engage the diaphragm and push the object on your stomach slightly higher.
- Slowly breathe out, again to a slow count. Pause at the bottom of the breath, then pull your stomach in a little bit more, toward your spine.

As you become more relaxed, increase the count to 4/8 (four counts on inhalation, eight counts on exhalation), then to 5/10, and up to 7/14 or 8/16. Stop if you feel dizzy or short of breath. Your breath should be strong, smooth, and uniform. If you sense restrictions in the flow of your breath, just continue to breathe through them and past them. Try not to gasp or sigh. Do this for two minutes each day.

You can also practice this on hands and knees. Keep your spine "in neutral," and belly breathe. This improves your ability to exhale with your abdomen, and makes you aware of how your diaphragm and breathing interact with your back muscles.

I'm confident that if you can start making these adjustments to your routine, you'll be more productive, feel more energetic, and waste less time at doctors' and therapists' offices. Cultivate and continue them as daily habits—for the rest of your life!

CHAPTER 3

Walk Before You Run

*If you can't fly, run. If you can't run, walk. If you can't walk,
crawl. But by all means, keep moving.*

—DR. MARTIN LUTHER KING JR.

MYTH: *We all know how to walk properly; there's nothing
much to learn.*

FACT: *Most of us walk incorrectly. Fortunately, proper form is
easy to relearn.*

MYTH: *Running makes you more fit than walking.*

FACT: *A consistent routine of walking results in increased
longevity and a level of overall health that is comparable to
what runners experience.*

For building fitness and health, many of us assume that running
is superior to walking. But increasingly, studies are reaching an
elementary conclusion: a consistent routine of *walking* is just as
good as running for preventing heart disease, type 2 diabetes,
Alzheimer's, and cancer. As a bonus, those who walk vigorously
and consistently enjoy improved cognitive function and mood,
and measurably lower mortality rates.

Surely there can't be a lot left to learn about the basic activity of walking. It's ridiculously simple—an instinctive movement,
requiring little thought. But there's a bit more to it than this. Surprisingly, most of us *don't walk correctly*. This isn't due to laziness or
a lack of training. But it *is* a by-product of our sedentary lifestyle.

Healthy walking can save your life in the long term. And for active-duty military, walking properly is essential to saving their lives in the short term. In 2015, I was invited to instruct a group of USAF Combat Controllers and parachute jumpers (PJs) on running form. As part of their training, these young Airmen jump out of planes, navigate "enemy" territory, and signal a target for an airstrike (this is usually done by someone on the ground). Then they have to get out alive.

I joined the trainees on a "ruck march" covering four miles at a clip of fifteen minutes per mile, with sixty pounds on our backs. These guys were master walkers, it turned out, and they made the march appear more like a morning stroll, despite the load and the pace. What these Airmen do so well, and with little thought, over thousands of miles, is what I'll attempt to describe below.

HOW DOES WALKING WORK, ANYWAY?

The mechanics of walking—the physiology and processes operating behind the scenes—rely on a complex choreography of muscles, fascia, joints, energy, balance, and volition. It's all dedicated to generating efficient forward motion, while protecting the body from injury.

The conscious brain deals with overall movement, not with individual muscles. If we had to intentionally direct every muscle in the process of walking, we would hardly be able to put one foot in front of the other. Instead, our myofascial tissues, which largely work at a subconscious level, react to triggers that originate in the brain, fascia, and muscles. These tissues have evolved to respond by loading tension on our joints and other tissues then releasing and redirecting that energy (like the springs of a trampoline) into forward movement.

Gravity is both our friend and our enemy. It pulls us down, but within that downward movement lies energy that can be harnessed as upward spring. Every surface that we travel over contains an inherent elastic spring, too. Compare the sensation of walking on soft sand with walking on a wooden floor. When you walk or run on a beach, much of the energy expended in each foot strike is dissipated into the sand (visualize the effort needed to compress and displace the sand in each footprint). By contrast, a wooden floor is far more elastic, storing the energy from your falling weight, then giving some of it back as you spring off the next step. The Harvard indoor track may be the perfect elastic surface—so good that running times recorded on it aren't allowed as certified records.

Take a look at a pendulum, as in a grandfather clock. With each swing through its arc, the pendulum's kinetic energy is at a maximum at the bottom of the swing. As it swings upward it slows, and this kinetic energy is converted to potential energy, reaching a maximum when the pendulum stops at the top of the swing. In a good-quality pendulum with a long arc, the conversion of energy back and forth from kinetic to potential is nearly 100 percent efficient.

Now picture the legs of a walking human as, quite simply, two pendulums. The kinetic energy of one leg is highest as the foot swings forward, at the bottom of the swing, and its potential (stored) energy is at its high point—fully loaded—when the foot is momentarily stopped and planted on the ground.

The efficiency of our dual leg pendulums, in freely carrying our movement forward, is only about 65 percent. This means that the additional 35 percent of the energy needed to complete each step (and keep moving) must come from the muscles. But there's room for improvement in walking efficiency. One study looked at Kenyan women who carry loads on their heads, and found that they shorten the midstance pause in their stride in order to minimize the energy dissipated into the ground. By converting more of their potential and kinetic energy into forward motion, they need less of a boost from their muscles (and expend fewer total calories of energy) than most of us would need to execute the same task. When carrying loads, energy conservation is at a premium, and the Kenyan women's efficiency of movement rises from 65 percent to as much as 80 percent.

HOW DOES THIS LOOK IN STOP-ACTION?

When we examine the mechanics of walking, how do the parts come together into this ordinary yet remarkable task?

Our joints and muscles don't work in isolation. We should

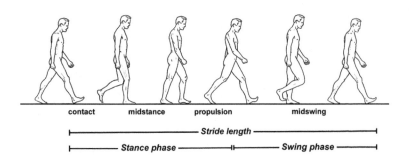

contact   midstance   propulsion   midswing

├──────────────── Stride length ────────────────┤

├──────── Stance phase ────────┤├──── Swing phase ────┤

think of the body as a complex array of parts linked tightly (and sometimes loosely) in a dynamic, interdependent, spring-loaded chain of movements. Let's dissect a normal walking stride.

The fleshy pad of the heel is the first part of the foot to strike the ground. Some of the ground impact energy is dissipated by this cushioning. The ankle joint absorbs impact next, followed by the knee, the hip, and finally the spine. The myofascial system, which provides balance and makes small corrections, also absorbs and dissipates much of the impact load, and stores some of that energy, too.

As the stride progresses, the landing leg becomes the trailing, toe-off leg, and the toes flex upward (dorsiflex), which resets and stabilizes the arch of the foot. At toe-off, the toes extend (causing plantar flexion of the ankle), the knee extends, the hip extends, the spine sways (or arches) slightly, and the soles point rearward and up.

WHERE DOES THE POWER AND SPRING COME FROM?

The supporting hip muscles (adductors, abductors, and glutes) must be strong, at the same time that the hip flexors (the group of muscles that includes the iliacus, psoas, and rectus femoris) must be long and mobile, for maximum backward leg extension from the hip joint. Tight hip flexors, and toes that don't readily dorsiflex (bend up), lead to a shortened stride.

Good locomotion depends on the strength and elasticity of our fascia and muscles during the push-off phase of the stride (when the foot is on the ground). Once the foot is airborne, it can't offer propulsion.

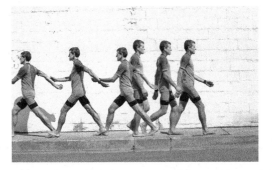

Tight hip flexors + stiff ball of foot + stiff shoes = short stride
Good mobility at hip and forefoot + flexible shoes = long stride

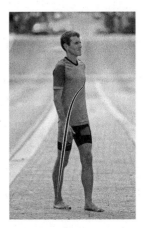

A short stride + minimal
counter-rotation of the shoulders
and pelvis + little hip extension =
weak spring

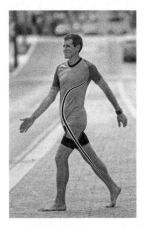

A long stride + good
counter-rotation of the shoulders
and pelvis + good hip extension =
powerful spring

There's another dynamic motion that occurs in walking: the shoulders counter-rotate (in the transverse plane) relative to the pelvis. This creates diagonal, springlike tension in an "X" across the front of the chest. With good hip extension, the tension and energy in this counter-rotation spring-loads the trailing leg for a rapid and efficient return to the front.

Now that we're up and walking, let's go through some simple adaptations we can make to improve the ease and efficiency of movement.

Posture, as we discussed in the previous chapter, is the best place to start in developing solid, efficient walking form. When your posture is good, your body's mass is supported by its *structure*, not by its muscles. If you suffer pain and fatigue from walking, or even from standing, this is the first clue that you have been using your muscles for balance, and that your posture is out of alignment. (A "museum stroll" is generally more tiring and less efficient, you might have noticed, than a power walk at higher speeds. This is because when you stroll, you are using the power of your muscles instead of the dynamic, load-and-spring feature of muscles and tendons, and are disrupting the rhythmic pendulum swing of the legs that occurs at a normal walking pace.)

Envision holding a garden rake with one hand from the end of its handle, the rake straight up in the air. When the rake is well balanced, it takes little effort to keep it in that position. But holding it even slightly out of alignment requires significant strength. It's the same with your spinal column. Shoes with elevated heels only exacerbate this postural misalignment.

DON'T BE UP THE STREET WITHOUT A PADDLE

The next time you walk, think of it as a new, mindful adventure.

Begin by straightening your frame so that it is tall, yet relaxed, and breathe from the diaphragm (as learned in the previous chapter). Gently lean forward from the ankles, and propel yourself into a walk. Think of your leg as a paddle that you place on the ground (the water), and by stroking it back it moves you (the canoe) forward.

Lead from the torso, not from the head. Maintain your gaze directly forward, not downward. As you walk, try this: place your hands on the front of your hips, and with each step make a conscious effort to leave each big toe on the ground for a split second longer than you usually would, and roll off of it as you push behind you. At the end of the stride, let the bottom of your foot turn up slightly—releasing the sole of your foot to be "tanned by the sun."

Your knee remains slightly bent on landing, but it fully extends on toe-off. Forward locomotion is all about the leg behind you, not the one in front. Pay attention to your powerful posterior muscles as they *press downward and behind you.* The trailing leg will naturally lift and bring itself forward. (The more extension you have behind you, the more readily your leg springs to the front.) As your hips open and your glutes activate, your stride will lengthen.

Let yours arms swing gently to and fro from the shoulders, like pendulums, with hands relaxed. Notice your feet. Your rounded heel works like a ball: it is designed to roll forward. As your weight shifts from heel to big toe, picture the mechanics of a wheel—one that smoothly rolls through the heel—rather than a jolting, sequential heel strike. Basic physics affirms that it is inefficient (and fatiguing) to walk by overextending your leg forward, locking your knee, and hitting the ground with a thud. Each step may not seem to land with much impact, but multiply that by two thousand per mile.

To follow all this and engage these subtle changes may feel strange at first, but your technique will become more fluid and natural as you progress. Walking will become gliding.

THESE SHOES ARE MADE FOR WALKING . . .

The principles that apply to running shoes (see the chapter on feet) apply to walking footwear as well. Your health care provider or shoe store may have told you to get a cushioned shoe with good arch support. But these narrow, soft, arch-supporting shoes only interfere with the function of your feet, disrupt your posture, and inhibit forward propulsion. In particular, elevated heels allow (and even encourage) a hard heel strike, triggering compensations in every joint from your ankle to the knee and hip, and up through the back. And arch supports block the natural, leaf-spring-like flattening of the foot. Some people complain of "fallen arches," but these are usually cases of *failing* arches—from years of disuse.

With practice and patience, the afflictions arising from modern shoes can almost always be reversed. Ernest Wood's *Zen Dictionary* states, "The foot feels the foot when it feels the ground." You will rediscover this connection, and the miraculous function of your feet, as you transition into thinner, flat, and more flexible shoes with a wide toe box and no arch support. Such minimalist shoes

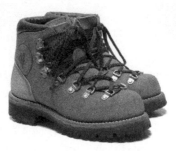

Remember these footwear bricks from a generation ago?
It's best to avoid hiking boots like these that don't allow a natural,
foot-to-ground connection.

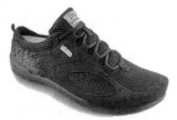

Shoes with wide toe boxes, and with no arch support or heel lift,
are ideal for walking. Elevated heels, common in modern
"cushy" running shoes, compromise foot balance and posture,
and encourage a hard heel strike.

allow your toes to spread apart and provide balance, and let your foot pronate and your arch flatten, then release locomotive power when they spring back.

I'm confident that once you progress (gradually) to wider- and thinner-soled shoes, you will never go back. But do talk to a knowledgeable health care provider if you have a structural or congenital condition that necessitates a supportive shoe.

Shoes with stiff, rocker-shaped soles—there are many of them—dampen natural energy return and generate instability as your foot rolls forward. The very front part of these (and most other) modern shoes curves slightly upward in what's called "toe spring," an intentional design feature that presumes that the foot needs help in "rolling" into the next step. But our toes were made to bend and flex and grip the surface of the earth. When shoes aim our toes toward the sky, our toes can't help us balance or propel. Ironically, the rocker shape also doesn't allow the toes to bend completely upward (dorsiflex) on toe-off—yet this is needed to create the stable platform that provides optimal propulsion.

It's fairly simple: we don't need shoes to try to do the foot's work for it. After all, the trial-and-error design features of our feet have evolved for a very long time. (The Laetoli footprints date to about 3.7 million years ago.)

My father had a hip replaced, and then a knee. During recovery, he was told that his other knee should be replaced, too. But before he signed up for surgery again, I convinced him to try modifying his walking technique, and to wear less substantial shoes. Three pairs of well-worn minimalist shoes later, he is walking and golfing pain-free, and has lost weight. He says that he feels great, with no hint of pain in the other knee. By realigning his posture, changing his walking technique, awakening the natural springs in his legs, and reducing impact on his joints, he added years of pain-free walking to his life.

KEEP ON TREKKIN'

If you need motivation to walk more, try some fun walking accessories. Heart rate monitors are a useful tool to keep track of your effort and your progressing fitness. Movement monitors (such as Fitbit) subtly challenge people to build a record of distance walked and number of steps taken. Try to increase your walking distance to five miles, or ten thousand steps a day. GPS watches can accurately measure distance, but your mobile phone likely has a free app that counts steps and logs distance traveled. Growing numbers of people swear by treadmill desks, and claim (once they are through the short learning curve) that they are more productive overall than when sitting at a desk.

When hiking or walking in the countryside, you may want to use Nordic poles. Hiking poles give more of your body a workout, and exercise the important "pulling" muscles of the shoulder (most exercise routines, and life activities, engage the pushing muscles). Many fitness programs mix running with walking, and I encourage this, too. As you quicken your cadence and lengthen your stride, your speed and heart rate will rise, and your cardiovascular system will benefit. Leki makes exceptional poles.

If you're too busy to dedicate time only to walking, then walk as you talk on the phone, or take someone with you. What's better than a roundtable discussion—a semispherical one in which you and your colleagues are surrounded, horizon to horizon, by the universe?

LET THE RETOOLING BEGIN

In the hospital, walking is the most important part of any post-surgical or disease recovery. Outside of a few unfortunate conditions such as spinal cord injury, the goal should always be to return quickly to walking efficiently and without pain. The principles of posture, balance, body awareness, hip extension, glute strength, and foot strength that we'll explore in the coming chapters apply equally to walking, and there is no safer or more accessible movement. Its natural flow, and the strength it builds, sets you up to experience relaxed and efficient running.

DRILLS

For sedentary people, walking is generally the safest (and easiest) way to start getting into shape. The initial prescription is quite simple: *Stand up and begin walking*. The next step: *Take the next step*. Repeat.

The next time you walk, try practicing these:

1. *Slow walk.* In bare or stocking feet, at home or on a smooth surface:
- Lengthen your spine (envision strings pulling you upward from the top of your head).
- Lean slightly forward from the ankles (imagine a gentle tug on the sternum).
- Land gently on your heel, but feel your weight quickly shift toward your midfoot, as your foot pronates and your toes splay outward.
- Push your foot *down and back* into the ground (the sensation of pushing along with one foot on a skateboard).
- Finish the stride with propulsion from all of your toes, and load the big toe especially. As your toes bend, your soles will almost turn upward (to be "tanned by the sun"). Your trailing leg will naturally spring forward.
- Listen to your foot strike. You should not hear a slap or a thud.
2. *Faster walk.* Notice that your degree of elbow bend affects your cadence (number of steps per minute).

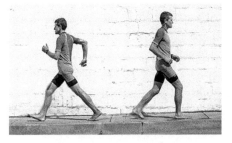

Fast walk versus slow walk

At a nice, relaxed saunter (window-shopping speed), your elbows will be straight and your cadence about fifty to sixty steps per minute. Now bend your elbows to about 45 degrees and watch your step count pick up to sixty to sixty-five per minute. For a real fitness walk, bend your arms to 90 degrees and drive the elbows back from the lower traps (the muscles at the bottom of the shoulder blades), which helps set the rhythm. Experiment. Everyone finds their own slightly different elbow angle that works for fastest, easiest walking.

3. *Stand and walk while you work.* If possible, work at a standing desk or even a treadmill desk. If you must sit, take every opportunity to stand up, walk, and stretch, such as when speaking with someone or talking on the phone. Ignore the looks of colleagues as you do lunges or swing a leg forward and back and from side to side. They'll get used to you.

4. *Walk barefoot in your home.* This strengthens your feet and lower leg tissues. Better yet, spend one day a week without shoes ("Barefoot Saturdays").

CHAPTER 4

The World Is Flat If You're a Foot

How one runs probably is more important than what is on one's feet, but what is on one's feet may affect how one runs.
—DR. DANIEL LIEBERMAN

MYTH: *Cushioned, supportive shoes of modern design protect your feet and your kinetic chain from injury.*

FACT: *There is no evidence that this is the case. Supportive shoes with elevated heels can even "disable" your feet by allowing them to fall out of shape, and can alter your body position and function, setting it up for injury.*

Let's take a look at the human foot. It's a physical adaptation—a biomechanical marvel—that is shared with no other primate. Even in medical school, I didn't fully learn about or appreciate the miraculous way it operates. Understanding how the foot functions by studying its anatomy alone is like trying to learn how a car works by examining its individual pieces.

The genius of the foot lies in the synchronized interaction of the joints, tendons, muscles, fascia, and nerves, and how they work in service to the rest of the body. This synchrony is controlled by the brain, the spinal cord, and even the local fascial tissue, which receives vital information about the terrain from thousands of nerve endings on the soles of the feet. When this sensing system is in harmony with its moving hardware, the foot becomes an unbeatable, self-sufficient, adaptable—living—machine.

The foot is also the least understood of the body's moving parts.

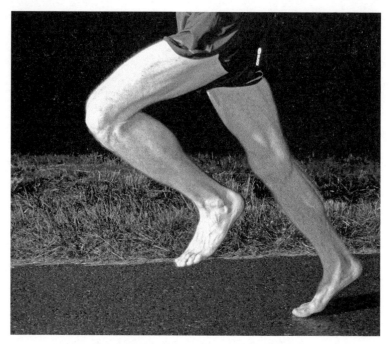

A partial view of the foot and lower leg. Every foot has
twenty-six bones, thirty-three joints, and more than a hundred muscles,
tendons, and ligaments, including the body's strongest, the Achilles tendon.
There are four layers of muscles in the soles of our feet alone.

In a basic sense, we do know that when force (mainly from gravity)
is applied to the foot, energy is dissipated and deflected through
the joints in several different directions. Indeed, the foot is perfectly built for its two most important functions: (1) shock absorption and (2) forward propulsion.

In addition to working like a shock absorber, the foot stores
much of the landing force of every step, then converts it to its
other essential function—forward motion. Here are a few of the
actions occurring simultaneously in a running foot as the weight
of the body falls on it:

- The plantar fascia is the ligament made of tough
  fibrous tissue that connects the heel to the base of the
  metatarsals, along the bottom of the sole. As more
  weight loads onto the foot, *the plantar fascia stretches*

and lengthens, absorbing shock and providing springlike recoil, like a leaf spring on a truck.
- *The foot pronates,* rolling from the outward edge inward, toward the big toe—dispersing impact in a sideways (inward) direction.
- The *toes splay outward,* adding balance and forward propulsion. The toes then dorsiflex (bend upward) and stabilize the foot for toe-off.

All of these motions—downward, to the side, and forward and back—dissipate the forces of impact at the same time that they create a wide, stable platform for the foot. Then, when the foot leaves the ground, the bending toes straighten to reset the plantar fascia and the transverse arch. The foot is cocked and ready for the next impact. Let's explore this.

THE ARCH AND THE WINDLASS

In engineering terms, the foot works like a windlass mechanism, in which the movement of one part transfers energy to another part, while initiating other compensatory movements. (Think of jetliner wheel assemblies, which are designed to trigger a cascading series of changes to the plane's behavior the moment the wheels touch the tarmac.) In the case of our foot, this complex ground contact response works with surprising efficiency.

At the moment when weight bears onto the forward leg, the foot is soft and flexible and acts as a shock absorber. Then the main, longitudinal arch flattens, stretching and "loading" the plantar fascia with stored energy, like a spring. (Place one foot lightly on the floor. Now place all your weight on it, and note how your toes move forward. This is your foot momentarily lengthening as the plantar fascia stretches and flattens.)

At the end of the running stride, this springlike energy is released like a slingshot, efficiently propelling you forward.

Try this: Reach down and pull your big toe upward. Watch the arch of your foot rise. You'll see this even if you have been told you have "flat feet."

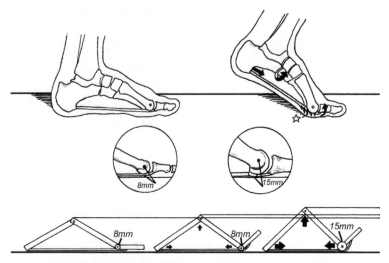

Picture the arch as a triangle. The plantar fascia ligament is at the bottom, and acts like a springy high-tension cable. At the completion of the stride, when the toes are bent upward, the plantar fascia shortens and tightens as it wraps beneath the metatarsal bones, elevating the arch.

PRONATION

Impact forces are also dispersed by *pronation*—the natural motion of the arch flattening as the foot rolls inward. This is best seen when running or landing from a jump, when the foot first contacts the ground on the outside edge, with the ankles tilted slightly outward. As the body weight settles onto the foot, the ankles roll inward and the foot flattens out.

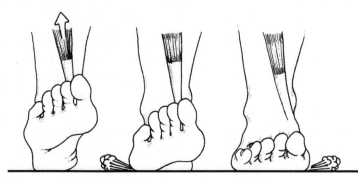

Pronation: the natural rolling from outward to inward.

Pronation dissipates a significant amount of shock. For this reason, despite its bad rap from the running shoe industry, it may be the most essential of all foot functions. Pronation can't occur naturally with arch supports or posted shoes. Many modern shoes, intending to protect us, block the foot from rolling inward. The impact forces are then relayed farther up the body into other structures that weren't designed to absorb the full impact.

TRANSVERSE ARCH FLATTENING

The ball of the foot is where five very mobile metatarsal bones are located. They are arrayed in an arch known as the *transverse arch*.

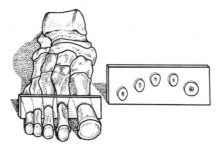

The second metatarsal acts as the keystone of the transverse arch.

With each step, the foot first connects with the ground on the outside, making for a soft touchdown for the landing foot. As body weight loads onto the foot, the transverse arch flattens like the springs in a suspension system. This widens the forward part of the foot, at the ball, by about 15 percent. This dynamic widening is rarely accounted for when shoes are being fitted, and is why you do *not* want a "snug fit."

EVEN THE TOES COME INTO (S)PLAY

As the five metatarsals flatten and widen on toe-off, the five toes want to splay even farther apart than the metatarsals, and reveal an open space between each toe. At this point, the lowly toes play a

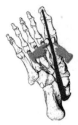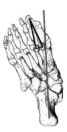

Correct alignment of the big toe (stable foot). Note the position of the sesamoids indicated by the fingers.

Alignment of the big toe with hallux valgus (unstable foot). Note the shift of the sesamoids.

vital role by (a) forming a stable, wide base of support, (b) giving feedback on the condition of the terrain in the form of sensory proprioception, (c) helping disperse the energy of impact, and (d) resetting the arch by tensioning the plantar fascia.

Normally the toes are the widest part of the foot. Unfortunately, since shoe design is dictated by fashion rather than by foot biomechanics, we mainly see shoes with tapered toe boxes. When the big toe—the captain of the ship—is not aligned, you are left with a foot that is unstable, is incapable of fully absorbing shock, and has limited propulsive properties. If you stand up and balance on one foot, you'll quickly understand the big toe's important stabilizing function. Can you feel it fully activated, gripping the ground?

I have a condition that is shared by millions of men and women called hallux valgus, a deformation of the big toe into a bent-inward position. This is typically caused by perpetually cramming our feet into the pointed toe boxes of most shoes (as I did when I was younger), and it is difficult to correct surgically. A product called Correct Toes can help by splaying and securing the toes in their normal anatomic position.

Twenty years ago, along with my hallux valgus, I suffered severe arthritis in my big toes. Surgery helped somewhat, but the Correct Toes almost immediately improved my balance and my stride efficiency. My feet again became magic springs, just as when I was a child running effortlessly on the beach. (I still wear the Correct Toes when I run, either in sandals or inside my shoes, as this condition has been difficult to fully correct.)

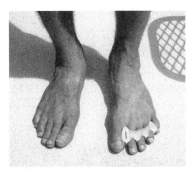

My foot. Note the inward angle of the large toe.

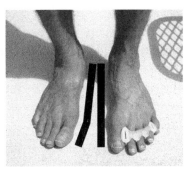

My foot with Correct Toes. Note that the big toe is properly aligned, in a straight line with the foot.

To see how this works, try the following:

- Place your feet squarely under your hips, and flare your toes as wide as you can. Think of the lunar lander.
- Hop as gently as you can, as if jumping rope, while maintaining a wide, stable foot position.
- Now squeeze your toes together and rotate your feet inward until they are in an overpronated position. Repeat the simple hops. Compare this more jarring *thud* to the earlier *boing, boing, boing* sensation.

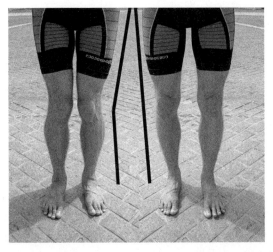

Weak, flattened feet (left) versus strong, springy feet (right). Note the effect on the alignment of the knees.

I share this digression on biomechanics with you for a simple reason: *the toes and plantar fascia ligament must be able to move freely, without restriction, for proper shock absorption and propulsion.* In its natural state (without shoes), the foot moves efficiently and safely. It rolls, stretches, expands, and grasps the ground. The role of a shoe should be to complement, and in some cases try to restore or re-create, *normal* foot function, while protecting us from the surface of the ground.

I frequently see adults in my store or medical clinic who are convinced they can no longer run. This is because they have allowed the natural springs in their feet and legs to be decommissioned, in effect, by improper footwear and by lack of use. When the natural springs of our feet are rendered ineffective, the joints end up taking the load. That load—the impact forces of running and walking, and the pain along with it—just gets shifted up the kinetic chain to our knees, hips, and spine. It's distressing to see this when we consider that the surface areas where each foot's thirty-three joints meet are large enough to dissipate the forces generated by a full lifetime of normal, unrestricted walking and running.

At least half of those who run suffer a running-related injury each year. In the U.S. military, lower-extremity-overuse injuries are a leading cause of lost days of duty—at a high cost to the taxpayer and to individual careers. This should not be the case.

SHOELESS BUT NOT CLUELESS

So, do we really need shoes? They do help us to endure extreme temperatures and to negotiate urban and off-road environments. But their precise function is still being debated.

Heavily cushioned footwear with arch supports, stability control, and elevated heels was introduced in the 1970s and became the norm in the 1980s. Gradually, shoe companies made them bigger and bulkier and snazzier—all to impart an illusion that they could improve performance and reduce injury. Common sense suggests that these contrivances would reduce impact between the (impossibly hard, unforgiving) pavement and our (delicate, injury-prone) feet.

Unfortunately, it has not worked out this way. Forty years later, there is no clinical or scientific evidence that cushioned, supportive shoes protect our feet and kinetic chain from injury.

How could this be?

It may be that the role of the shoe has been misunderstood. The modern, comfortable, cushioned shoe was designed as a solution to a problem that was never clearly defined. It was intended to compensate for *perceived* weaknesses and hazards. In one sense, these shoes have eased the burden on our feet so that they need to work less. But our feet are designed to work hard. In doing work, they gain strength. Our ancestors did not have golf courses.

A shoe's most important function should be to protect our soles, the same way that work gloves protect our hands. Beyond that, they should *allow our feet to behave like feet,* with freedom and flexibility, so that the muscles can rebuild strength and natural springiness. Along the way, they will be better protected from injury.

In particular, elevated heels—a feature of most modern footwear, including running shoes—shift the center of mass forward and away from the critical site in the foot that is meant to bear load (the sustentaculum tali, for medical folks). When the heel is elevated, the arch is destabilized, and the fifth metatarsal (another key stability structure) is lifted off the ground. This causes a domino effect of compensations. Abnormal forces are generated in our knees, hips, and lower back, as we alter our natural standing, walking, and running posture.

Make a short stack of wooden building blocks. Now slightly elevate one edge of the block at the bottom of the stack. To restabilize the stack, you'll need to slightly adjust the position of every block. Picture how this is routinely being done to your feet, knees, hips, and spine. (I'll readily grant that if you have a bit of heel elevation and are running pain free, I wouldn't insist you should change shoes.)

UNEXPECTED CONSEQUENCES

Shoes with motion-control features, which restrict pronation, are potentially injurious. One study found that U.S. military trainees may have suffered *higher* injury rates in shoes that were prescribed

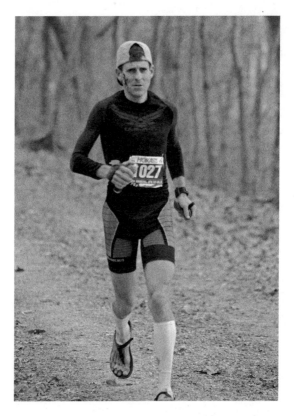

The 2016 JFK 50 Mile run, in Shamma Sandals and Correct Toes

specifically for their perceived foot types. In particular, "rocker toes" don't allow the toes to fully dorsiflex, and they inhibit the arch from fully resetting itself at the end of the stride. If you combine this with an elevated heel and a narrow toe box, your muscles, tendons, and ligaments will shorten and weaken over time, and your default posture will change.

Soft cushioning of the heels and soles presents another problem, by encouraging a long, bounding stride, accompanied by heel striking. In a thinner, less cushioned shoe, overstriding is uncomfortable, and you naturally avoid doing it. Thinner shoes also offer more proprioception, or sensory feel for the ground. If you can sense the terrain beneath you, the muscles in your feet and core fire more quickly and decisively, helping to stabilize you and improve running efficiency, while building strength in your feet. We will discuss overstriding in chapter 8, on mobility.

When I was first injured in high school track, I was told to run in *supportive* shoes. And when I was *re*injured, I was advised to run in *supportive shoes with an orthotic*. I did this for years, until I started to notice something: my legs' elastic springs weren't being called on to perform. They grew weaker and less resilient. As my athletic bag filled with orthotics and other shoe accessories, my condition worsened as my spring dampened. Five years of chronic plantar fasciitis (and debilitating large-toe pain) later, in the year 2000, I finally had surgery.

Surgery helped, but not as much as better running form and less substantial shoes. I started by cutting off the heels of my cushioned shoes, and removed the inserts. I have since completed more than fifty marathons (and multiple ultra-marathons) in such minimalist shoes.

SO, WHAT'S THE BEST SHOE?

In the running world, the subject of shoe design has become divisive and political, with an abundance of claims and counterclaims, all supported by sketchy science. We need to hurdle over the shoe and running rhetoric and ask what kinds of shoes enhance the natural biomechanics of the foot and protect and strengthen the kinetic chain. A shoe should complement nature, not try to outsmart it.

The array of athletic footwear for sale is bewildering. Fortunately, there are now many brands and styles of shoe that simply *let our feet be feet*. No single shoe is perfect for everyone, and no single shoe may be perfect even for one person. But through a few simple assessments, readers should be able to make an educated choice of what can work best for their bodies relative to their running environments. Each of us is an experiment of one, and we should expect some trial and error in the shoe selection process.

There are some basic elements of shoe design, however, that work to enhance natural foot function:

- A flexible sole. The shoe should bend easily and allow the foot to flex and expand and contract naturally. (The more flexible the sole, the stronger your foot needs to be, too.)

- A lower "drop"—or no drop—in elevation from heel to toe. This is the difference in height between the heel and the forefoot, and can be thought of as the slope or grade. Modern shoes typically have a 6 to 10 percent grade, and we know what that means on the highway: caution! If the shoes you are accustomed to wearing (whether athletic or street shoes) have elevated heels, reduce the height of the heels, especially for standing and walking. Information on drop, in millimeters, is available for many athletic shoes.
- A thinner shoe. If your running shoes have thick, soft soles, look for a shoe that allows you to feel more of the ground (which will help train you away from overstriding). It takes more energy to walk or run on a soft surface—think sandy beach. You want a firm surface to act as a platform to set your stride. Thinner shoes are also lighter, a huge bonus for overall comfort and efficiency.

Select shoes based on fit, not size. You need plenty of room for your toes to splay and your feet to stretch as they move. When sized properly, you may end up in a shoe a full size or two larger than what you had before.

TRANSITIONING TO MINIMALIST

Moving to lower-drop or minimalist footwear should be a process, not an event. The muscles, tendons, and ligaments in your feet and legs need time to lengthen and strengthen. While adapting a little soreness is inevitable but you should not be in pain.

Few people can run in ultra-minimalist Vibram FiveFingers right away, but you can start walking and playing in a minimalist shoe immediately. Walking is the perfect transition. Or try "transition shoes"—an intermediate pair (or two) that gradually introduce you to the features just listed. Such transition shoes typically have 4 to 6 millimeters of drop (elevation loss from heel to toe), versus the standard 12 to 14 millimeters of drop in most running shoes.

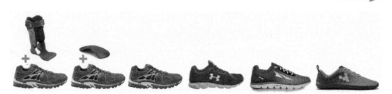
Gradually reduce your support, and rediscover spring in your step.
Progression can take months to years.

Begin by going barefoot as much as possible—at home, for instance—and wear your minimalist shoes for work and for walking, as these activities involve less impact. Mix it up!

When you begin to master the art of slow, comfortable jogging, with a short, rhythmic stride and quicker cadence, you'll be using muscles and tendons the way they were designed. Your feet will tend to land less on the heel—which is good, because heel landings slow you down like a brake, and deliver jarring forces. You'll naturally land more on the midfoot. Count on three to twelve months to rebuild the strength and flexibility that modern shoe designs have taken away from you. It may take five years to build up to running a marathon in sandals.

There's a bonus to wearing lighter footwear, too. British researchers measured higher oxygen consumption (energy expenditure) by runners wearing shoes, compared to running in bare feet. They attribute this to the additional energy needed to carry the mass of the modern shoe. (The effect of any weight on the lower legs is magnified when compared to carrying the same weight closer to the core.)

Most runners find little long-term help from podiatrists and other medical specialists, and instead seek advice and share experiences at their local running hangout. My store, Two Rivers Treads in Ranson, West Virginia, has become a running and footwear clinic—an informal laboratory for assessing and understanding runners' problems. We make a point of offering only advice and education that is evidence-based and truly useful. The process has been fascinating: the customers, and the runners in the local races, have taught me more than I have taught them.

IT'S NOT ONLY ABOUT THE FEET

If I sound like an advocate trying to steer you away from the mainstream, then believe me: if you are already running joyously, without pain, stick with what you have. Even if you are not injured, however, you may want to move to a more minimalist shoe and see how your feet and your body respond. You might be surprised.

The feet are just the beginning: the impact forces of running are so great that they must also be absorbed by the legs, hips, and back—all the way up the body's kinetic chain. At each point along this chain, those forces are sensed, absorbed, stored, and released in similarly miraculous and interconnected ways. We'll explore this dynamic biomechanical progression in the chapters to come.

DRILLS

Our goal is to develop internal strength, coordination, and support for the muscles of the feet. As my colleague Jay Dicharry puts it, "You need less from your shoes, more from you." To determine if you're ready for minimalist running, you may want to watch the video (on the book website's videos page) that Dicharry and I shot for *Running Times*. And if you've been wearing highly supportive or confining footwear, the drills in this chapter offer a plan for making the transition.

Foot posture
- *Toe yoga*. Stab your entire big toe down to the ground, while lifting the other four. Bend only at the metatarsophalangeal (MTP) joint (see arrows in the images below), without curling the toes. Now lift the big toe while stabbing the other four down. Your arch will naturally rise. Repeat. This helps develop foot control.

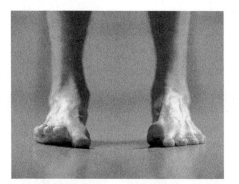

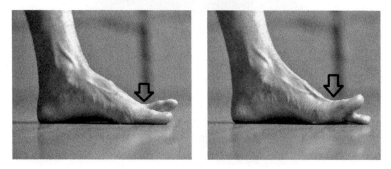

- *Short foot posture.* Create a "dome" by elevating your arch and anchoring (not curling) your toes, while driving the first metatarsal head to the ground. (See the "Short Foot Posture" video at runforyourlifebook.com.) This effectively shortens your foot, and it involves moving your knees just slightly to the outside—from a slightly knock-kneed stance to a straight stance. (If you move your knees any farther, you would appear bowlegged. Refer to the images below.)

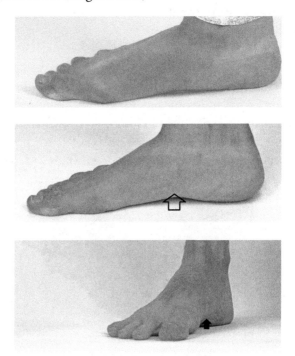

To realign your feet, repeat the foot posture exercises above whenever you can throughout the day—at work, in class, while standing in line, even while brushing your teeth.
Within a few weeks, your base of stability will improve.

- *Slow heel raises.* While balancing on your right foot (use a hand to secure yourself, if needed), slowly lift your heel so that you are balancing on the ball of your foot. Go up as high as you can, then rotate your lower leg slightly counterclockwise, as your weight naturally transfers to the big toe. This is the same rotation that occurs in your lower leg at the end of the running stride, as power shifts to the big toe for toe-off. Then slowly lower yourself. Do the same with your left foot, rotating your lower leg just slightly clockwise at the top of the lift. Do this up to fifty times on each foot, once or twice a day (at your stand-up desk!), and you'll see greatly improved foot control.

- If you would like to transition to more minimalist shoes and techniques, try *a small amount of barefoot running*. There are about twelve hundred steps in one mile of running, but even running a hundred yards down the sidewalk and back will give you quality, outdoor exercise for your feet. Early experiments with barefoot running should be done on a safe, smooth, firm surface, while listening to your body. Run slowly but at a high cadence, with a soft, springy motion (not bounding). Your forward speed may be slower than a fast walk. It's okay if your feet are a bit sore the next day, but you should not experience pain. Progress gradually. This may seem difficult, but it should also make you smile. After months and years, you will have bulletproof, resilient feet.

- *Light hopping drills and jumping rope* awaken the springs of the feet. Many of these simple drills—part of the U.S. Air Force Phase One Drills series of exercises—can be viewed on the book website's videos page.

CHAPTER 5

The Springs That Move Us

There are those who suffer and grow strong; there are those who suffer and grow weak. This mystery of pain is still for me the saddest of earth's disabilities.

—SILAS WEIR MITCHELL, *doctor and patient*

MYTH: *Structurally, the body functions mainly through the interaction of muscle and bone, with some involvement of tendons and ligaments.*

FACT: *The connective tissue known as fascia (which includes tendons and ligaments) plays a much larger role than we ever imagined in how our bodies work.*

MYTH: *Running mainly requires strength.*

FACT: *Running requires "spring" as much as strength.*

My own discovery of the fluidity, grace, abounding energy, and injury-free comfort that can result from smooth running form didn't happen immediately.

After a lot of trial and error (including serious pain avoidance and suppression), I gradually learned how to judiciously pace my running, how to harness my body's internal springs, and how *not* to land a step. The more that I discovered and understood this, the more I trended toward wearing minimal shoes and tending to my fascia—and the better I felt.

Our muscles, tendons, bones, nerves, and internal organs are all suspended and sheathed in a web of connective tissue known as *fascia*. This collagenous material begins a couple of millimeters below the level of our skin, and permeates our bodies, appearing variously as stringy clumps, as closely packed bundles, and as layers of mats, sheets, and films. Some of it is delicate, some tough and fibrous. Some of it binds structures together, while some lubricates the organs so that they smoothly glide over each other in order to dissipate (or relay) the mechanical forces generated by the muscles. In essence, the fascia facilitates everything that moves in our bodies, in an efficient, coordinated way.

When you dissect a wedge of orange, you expose progressively smaller, individually wrapped cells filled with juice. Everything but the raw, liquid juice itself is formed of connective tissue. This is comparable to the fascia in our bodies.

Surgeons tend to regard fascia as the nondescript, light-colored stuff that they slice through en route to the muscles, bones, or internal organs they've targeted. Fascia is omitted from the anatomical charts on the walls of your doctor's office, in order to better display these other organs. But it's the fascia that encases and suspends them all. It even cushions the spaces between our vertebrae (our discs are a form of fascia). Ligaments (a type of fascia) join bone to bone, while tendons (another type of fascia) join muscle to bone.

So how does fascia work, relative to our muscles and bones? Its operation can be illustrated in an unusual way.

TENSEGRITY: TENSION AND INTEGRITY

Our musculoskeletal system is conventionally viewed as individual muscles acting upon bones. But this doesn't fully explain our remarkable ability to move gracefully and efficiently over long distances on two legs, while maintaining near-perfect balance.

The skeleton is not a stack of bones, like building blocks sitting atop each other. You might have seen that medical school skeletons are held together with wires. That's because in life the bones mostly float independently—wrapped and swathed in layers of fascia. We would collapse in a heap without this connective tissue.

Some highway bridges, such as the iconic Golden Gate Bridge,

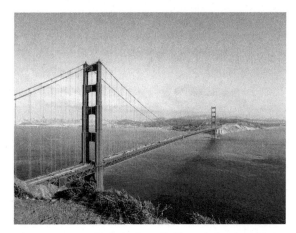

Tensegrity structures gain their strength through the dynamic interplay of tension and compression. The Golden Gate Bridge

are constructed according to a flexible, dynamic design principle known as *tensegrity*, or tensional integrity. They are strong and stable, yet dynamic, built on the interplay of tension and compression. Traditional suspension bridges employ some of these design features, modern designs even more.

First defined by Buckminster Fuller in the 1960s, tensegrity also describes the relationship between our bones (the struts) and the muscles, ligaments, tendons, and other fascia (the connecting cables), as seen in the models below. Bones provide great compressive strength, while muscles and fascia provide continuous tension, all in a strong, tightly linked yet flexible matrix.

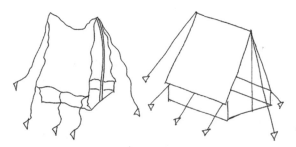

Like a tent, the fascia brings optimal integrity to the structure only when it is fully tensioned.

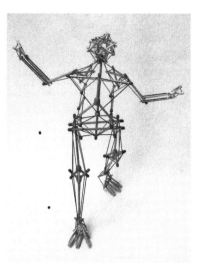

To a surprising degree, the dynamic structure of our bodies and the interplay of its parts work on these same principles of tensegrity.

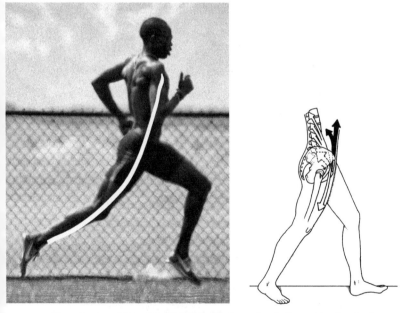

Olympian Lopez Lomong loads his hip flexor fascia (traced by the line). The more tension he creates through powerful propulsion and hip extension, the swifter his leg springs forward.

BOUNCE BACK BETTER

If left unattended (think prolonged sitting), the fascia grows slug-gish and stiff, and will constrict the muscles and the nerves. Many people don't realize that (over a period of several months) the elas-tic properties of the body's myofascial tissues can change. There is a term in materials science called *elastic hysteresis,* which is com-monly illustrated with a simple rubber band. If you apply force or load to the band, it stretches (deforms)—but returns much of that loaded energy when the force is withdrawn. A super-bouncy ball is said to have a tight elastic hysteresis curve (when the ball is thrown to the ground, little energy is lost between loading and the return bounce), whereas a hacky sack or Nerf ball has a very fat elastic hysteresis curve (there is little bounce—almost all of its energy is lost).

By training and minding our fascia, we can significantly tighten the elastic hysteresis curve of our fascia and enhance its springiness and energy. Children exemplify this: they can hop like kangaroos or jump rope for hours. Throughout, their calf muscles are mainly used isometrically, for stabilization and balance. The length of the muscle fibers changes little. The lengthening and spring and bounce in their legs comes primarily from the fascia:

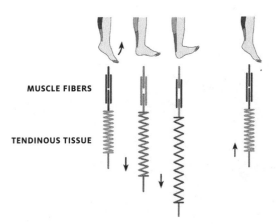

MUSCLE FIBERS

TENDINOUS TISSUE

When running well, muscle length changes only minimally.
Most of the movement and bounce occurs in the fascia, especially
the tendons and connective tissue.

For an impressive example of how to train this, watch "Ethiopian Runners Training Off-Season" on the videos page of runforyourlifebook.com and see the rhythmic plyometric drills of Ethiopian runners exercising during the off-season.

THE TRICKS PLAYED BY PAIN

All of this movement and tension is healthy for the fascia—up to a point. The collagen fibers of the fascia must slide, flex, and stretch smoothly in order to work properly. The fibers, which are normally arranged in springy waves or interwoven nets of tissue, flatten out as they withstand great unidirectional tension.

But when the fascia is *overly* stressed, it can become bunched into a knot, and we quickly become aware of it: the fascia is densely arrayed with receptors and nerve endings that telegraph pain and discomfort. It's like yanking hard on the ends of a rope to untangle a knot: it only makes the knot harder and tighter. Too often, we do exactly this in the name of physical therapy and traditional stretching exercises.

Only recently has the medical community begun to realize how important all this connective tissue is to the efficient, pain-free movement of our bodies. Among runners, fascial microtears and inflammation (such as Achilles tendinosis, iliotibial or IT band syndrome, and plantar fasciitis) comprise most of the chronic ailments and nonspecific recurring pain that I see. Almost every runner (and countless walkers) have experienced plantar fasciitis (or more accurately fasciosis) at some point in their lives.

In order to seek relief from the pain and while hoping to avoid future injury, we often focus on the place that hurts, though the restriction that was causing the pain may have originated at some distance from the injury. With plantar fascia pain, which originates in the sole of the foot, we often need to loosen the Achilles tendon and do some deep squats to open up the hip flexors, which tighten and shrink when we sit for long periods.

Many doctors are stumped by patients who complain of pain that originates in the fascia, because it's not readily visible in X-rays or on MRIs or CT scans. But growing numbers of sports physicians and physiotherapists have developed a deep understanding of it, and they use their eyes and hands as their primary diagnostic tools.

It is now believed that even psychological stress can contribute to fascial injuries; the fascia tightens and hardens in response to emotional and mental stimuli, predisposing one to injury.

THE CARE AND FEEDING OF YOUR FASCIA

No one feels loose and springy when they first wake up in the morning. It takes ten to twelve minutes of exercise for our bodies to warm up, as the fascia loosens and melts the sticky stuff in the intermuscular spaces. (Picture a cat stretching when it arises from a nap.) When we immobilize a joint or remain in a fixed position for an extended period, the synovium-lubricated fibrous web of cartilage and collagen (fascia) that encases the joint capsules becomes sludgy and stuck together. Sticky microadhesions then form between fascial surfaces, and harden sufficiently to inhibit our range of motion. Over time (within as little as a week in the case of a shoulder), this immobilization can cause "freezing" of the joint. The shoulder can be "melted" and the stuck fascia restored to its range of motion, but usually not without pain and extensive work. Unfreezing a joint sometimes requires heavy sedation.

WORK IT ON OUT, NOW

Imagine stretching a piece of taffy. This is your fascia. We tend to assume that the thin areas (where the injuries occur) are the sites that need to be treated. But movement and manipulation of the stuck-together bunched areas, which may be remote from the injury site, *fills in* the thinner, injured areas. Injured plantar tissue in the sole of the foot, for instance, usually requires loosening and stretching around the bunched areas in the feet, hips, and ankles. This is what the foam roller and other fascia work does.

The process of restoring flexible, strong, and resilient fascia can take between six months and two years. Be patient. While doing these exercises, move and stretch slowly, holding and "relaxing into" the stretches, because the fascia responds more slowly than muscles do. Fascial fitness training is not a substitute for strength work, endurance training, or improvement of form, but it is an important element of a healthy training program.

At my store in West Virginia, we do simple corrections to runners' and walkers' gaits almost daily. We start the runner off with some soft-tissue foam rolling, then have them open the hips with a few Mountain Climbers, and then move to the Awesomizer, all described below. In most cases, the runner's stride visibly opens—lengthens—and he or she starts to engage the powerful glute muscles. Nothing else out there is as powerful as this progression for bringing immediate change.

1. *Foam roll* the "knots." First thing every morning, take a few minutes to fully stretch out, head to toe. Then with a foam roller, "tissue floss" by rolling your legs, hips, torso, and back—gently and slowly—while remembering to breathe from the diaphragm. Your body will tell you where it needs attention. Roll from the middle of the muscle group up to its insertions, while avoiding the joints. When you find an area of tightness or tension, slowly roll out the knots by massaging above and below the area, for at least ten to fifteen seconds. (Ageless track phenomenon Olga Kotelko, the subject of the book *What Makes Olga Run?*, used a wine bottle as a foam roller.)

   You are rolling not just fascia but also muscles, nerves, and other connective tissue. Picture squeezing a sponge, then allowing it to fill again with water. Squeeze out the stiffness and congestion, and allow relaxation and fluidity to flow into the voids.

   The calf region is especially prone to restriction, and needs regular attention. Those who sit for hours (locked in that familiar forward flex) should focus on the hip flexors and upper back. An area often neglected is near the ASIS (the anterior superior iliac spine, a bony projection of the iliac bone) and the PSIS (posterior superior iliac spine). And foam roll areas adjacent to the

IT band and the quads, which often have adhesions. While lying on the floor on your side, you can slide your hips over a foam roller.

Mix up the areas that you foam roll each day. Be slow and mindful. This is not a rushed activity performed while answering emails or texts.

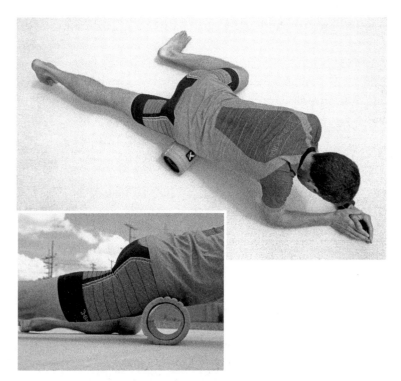

Rolling the ASIS (anterior superior iliac spine)

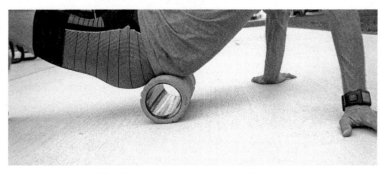

Rolling the PSIS (posterior superior iliac spine)

2. *The Mountain Climber* is remarkably effective at opening up and releasing your hips, as well. It can be done before a run or a walk or after an activity—or anytime, really.

Place your hands and feet on the ground, as in the illustration below, with your right foot to the outside of your right hand. Sink your left hip by squeezing the glute. Shift and move the position of the back leg by rotating your foot (lean your heel to the outside and then to the inside). When you move it to the outside, it helps open the IT band, and to the inside it stretches the inner thigh. Switch feet and repeat. Don't forget to sink the hips. Once you've loosened up, you can go dynamic and spring from one foot up to the other.

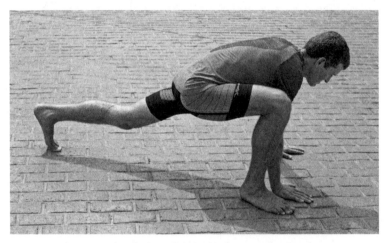

The Mountain Climber: Sink the hip by engaging the glute.
Feel the spring from the hip flexors.

3. *The Awesomizer*. Developed by Dr. Lawrence van Lingen, the Awesomizer is one of the easiest and most effective ways to release tightened hip flexors and tune the fascia of your pelvis and legs—all the way down to your feet.

- Stand and face a chair or low wall, about three feet from it. A solid table can work.
- Place your feet shoulder-width apart, so they point directly to the wall.

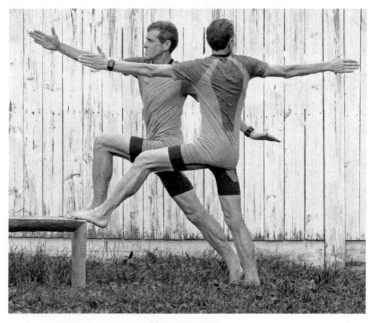

The Awesomizer

- Place your right forefoot on the wall, directly in front of it. (Before you do this, rotate your shoulders very slightly to the right and look at the spot where the right foot will go. This closes the hip and puts it in a position of power.)
- Keeping your rear (left) foot straight, rock back on your left foot and release your right hamstring.
- Lunge gently into the wall (lead from the hips) and rotate to the right, closing the hips. Feel the spring tension in the hip flexors.
- Rock back and rotate to the left, opening the hips. You should feel a release on your inner thigh.
- Repeat on the other side.

In addition to tuning your fascia, this movement will bring balance and relaxation to your walking and running stride. You can view some adjustments and "accessories" to Dr. van Lingen's "Awesomizer," on the videos page of runforyourlifebook.com.

4. *The dynamic burpee* is a bit more advanced. This exercise, created in the 1880s, is a combination of a squat, push-up, and jump, and is the ultimate full-body fascia exercise. It requires significant flexion and extension, and when it is done well you can feel the body dynamically spring off the ground.

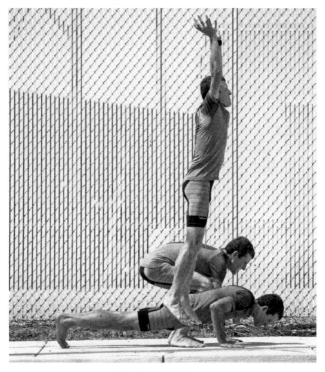

The dynamic burpee

- From a standing position, drop to a squat and place your hands on the ground (flexion).
- Transition into a push-up (with slight extension in the back).
- Quickly move back up to a squat (flexion).
- Jump up to finish (extension and reach).

When this exercise is done well, you should feel more spring and less power. Start with just a couple of repetitions, then progress to a few sets of six to eight. You don't need to do many—they're meant to be done skillfully, not to exhaustion.

5. *The couch stretch.* Perfect for stretching the rectus femoris, while loosening the hip flexors. Start with your foot against a wall or couch, then progress to holding your own ankle.

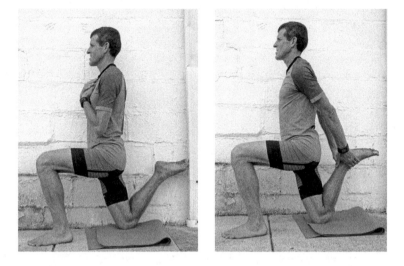

6. *Other techniques for tuning the fascia* may be helpful, such as fascial unwinding, yoga, Rolfing, the Alexander Technique, and the Feldenkrais Method. Soft tissue therapy may be needed for tough areas. The science and application of IASTM (instrument-assisted soft tissue mobilization) are also advancing.

7. Most important, here are *some simple tips for keeping your fascia healthy*, and for building the sensation of comfortable, fluid movement:

- *Stay hydrated.* Like the rest of the body, fascia is composed mainly of water.
- *Eat healthy fats.* Fats are the magic silicone that lubricates the moving cables, which you want to keep well "oiled."
- *Maintain movement* and mobility throughout the day. Stretch and lengthen in the morning and after sitting, and do multidirectional lunges.
- *Warm water is magic.* Soaking in a hot tub or warm bath

can loosen tight fascia, and muscles, too. Follow the bath with gentle mobility to restore any range of motion lost during the day. If you have access to a hot tub, stretch while relaxing in the water.

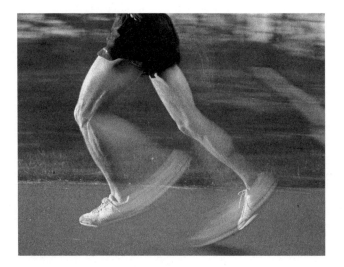

Finding time to work these and other routines into our modern daily lives may seem like a daunting challenge. But with creativity, and a few moments set aside, you may be able to incorporate many of these movements into your routines of work and play and domestic life. Once we have tuned up our magically springy fascia, it doesn't take much to maintain its elasticity throughout our lifetimes.

PART II

The Body in Motion

CHAPTER 6

The Elements of Style

Whether it's your golf score, your time on a two mile run, your soccer team's goals—everybody's looking at numbers. But they are not looking at the fundamentals.

—GRAY COOK, physical therapist

MYTH: *Running damages the joints. If you suffer pain, stop running.*

FACT: *Running isn't the problem—it's how you run. Adopt a low-impact, balanced, consistent technique and rhythm, and progress gradually.*

Most sedentary people view running as arduous and uncomfortable, regardless of how it's done. Accomplished runners, too, routinely complain of going from painful injury to painful injury. Too many of those who do run become frustrated or resigned to their fate—or they quit altogether.

Running isn't the problem. It's *how* we run. There are ways to run that generate suffering and injury, and there are other ways to run that bring health and a sense of joy. Except in unusual instances—severe degenerative disease, joint deformities, or rare medical cases that restrict activity—running is not only possible but distinctly beneficial.

Understandably, repetitive stress injuries occur more frequently from running than from walking. When running, each stride generates a momentary impact force nearly three times our body weight. Any imbalances or imperfections in our form are then amplified by twelve hundred of these poundings every mile.

The best way to address this is to develop a low-impact, consistent technique and rhythm, and progress gradually. I hope that you can discover, as I did, that seemingly subtle changes in running form can make a profound difference in how you feel, and can reduce your risk of injury.

FORM IS FUNCTION

The cardiovascular system, as we've learned, can be compared to a hybrid motor vehicle engine. When it's in tune, it can power you efficiently over long distances and provide quick accelerations for steep hills. But the chassis, shock absorbers, steering, linkage, and drive train are important, too. If your posture is out of alignment and your form is flawed, the risk of excessive wear and tear to the body's biomechanical parts increases.

Good running form is easy to learn. You don't need to study kinetics or kinematics, or submit to complicated, tedious drills. At the outset, simply observe how children run. Notice how they stand—balanced and erect, tall and straight—and how they move and leap with light steps and a springing motion. Their arms are bent. They don't overstride. Their overall movements are characterized by a sense of play, like improvisational dance. This may seem like an odd approach to running, but relearning this natural movement (and unlearning bad habits and misconceptions) requires that we start by imitating kids.

FIVE PRINCIPLES

Let's put what we've learned in the preceding chapters to work, and engage these five basic principles of good running form:

- The *first principle* is to *maintain proper posture*. Run tall. Think of your body as a straight, vertical line. Keep your neck straight and your head from drooping forward.

Look straight ahead, toward the horizon. Plant your feet flat on the ground. This is your neutral posture—the position of balance and strength. As you naturally begin to run, maintain this tall, neutral posture, and gently move your head slightly forward—as if stepping in to kiss someone. Many runners get stuck in a shoulder-forward and bent forward position, pulled by the dominant muscles in the front (the pecs and deltoids) and tight upper trapezius muscles. You can "reset" these by loosening the chest, then activating the lower traps by settling your shoulder blades—as if returning quick-draw pistols to their holsters.

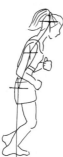 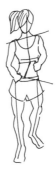

Improper alignment

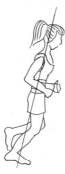 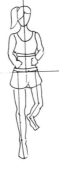

Proper alignment

- Now that you are running, the *second principle* is to *maintain a strong and stable core,* which includes your abdominals, pelvis, hip stabilizers, glutes, and even your shoulders. Visualize a can of compressed air in your belly.

Hunching over inhibits your breathing, deflating the can. In movement, this is your *dynamic posture,* and it demands that the parts of your neuromuscular system (brain, nerves, and muscles) work together seamlessly. Strong and active abdominal muscles and diaphragm, and stable hips, allow for the greatest energy transfer to and from the ground. This positions the joints correctly to deal with the loads, and causes the least stress on joints and muscles. Your knees should not collapse toward the midline of your body. Remain stable but relaxed.

- The *third principle* of good running form is to *use your arms and hands to set your rhythm.* Keep your elbows at an angle of 90 degrees or less, and drive the elbows back with the strong muscles of the lower trapezius and shoulders—but in a relaxed manner, such that your arms reflexively come forward. Your knuckles stay close to your sternum, but should not cross your center line. Think of chicken wings. The swing of the arms helps in four ways, by:

  - *providing stability*
  - *counterbalancing the movement of the opposite leg*
  - *balancing the pelvis*
  - *helping maintain forward momentum*

  Your shoulders provide a gentle rotation that is counter to your lower body, too. In effect, you are "winding up" with a twist. This loads the fascia and adds more spring to your step.

- The *fourth principle* of good running form is to *ensure that your feet actively moderate the impact.* Each foot should land with the full foot making contact at a position to load the spring and not the brake. Avoid overstriding or landing with a straight knee and foot stretched out in front. A full-foot landing pattern maintains balance, reduces shock, decreases the risk of injury, and is more efficient. Don't be overly concerned about which part of your foot lands first: it's all in where and how the landing forces are absorbed. Imagine the lunar lander: part of your foot touches the surface a little bit in front, part to the rear, but most of the force is straight down. And when you land with the knees slightly bent, you are set up for a stronger response by the muscles when you toe off in the next step. This should be visualized (and felt) as loading a powerful spring that helps launch the next step.

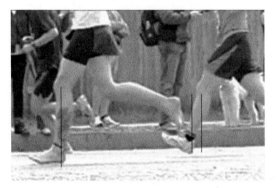

The barefoot runner on the left (in the Boston Marathon) isn't overstriding. His lower leg lands perpendicular to the ground, and his foot is evenly weighted on landing. The runner on the right has an outstretched lower leg and dorsiflexed ankle—characteristics of overstriding.

- The *fifth principle* of good running form is *cadence, or rhythm*. Efficient, springy runners maintain a cadence close to 180 steps per minute—regardless of the terrain or steepness, up or down. Find the rhythm that best harnesses the energy from your springs. Feel how some of the ground impact force is returned to you, especially when firing from the glutes (which produces a "pop" off the ground, in the manner that a pogo stick recoils). This motion shouldn't be viewed as actively *lifting* your leg. The recoil *sends* your leg forward and upward, on its own, like a slingshot. This is elastic recoil.

  The elastic recoil of your legs tends to become optimal as your cadence approaches 180 steps per minute, or three steps per second. Find what feels natural for you. Though your *cadence* remains fairly constant, your *stride length* may change. Your stride will be shorter at slow speeds and on uphill stretches, longer at faster speeds and on downhill sections. Adjust your stride and cadence to a

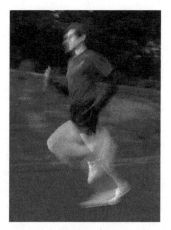

Run tall with a strong core. The arms are relaxed, elbows bent.
Lead from the hips and power from the glutes.
Top it off with a soft, full-foot landing and natural rhythm.

pace at which you can hold a conversation. Most increase cadence at faster speed. The cadence that most people fall into tends to be slightly slower than what is optimally efficient, as measured in the lab. Metro Timer and Pro Metronome are two free apps that can help.

SLOW JOGGING

Most of those in the military with whom I work admit that they hate running. But when I frame it as "slow jogging" and get them

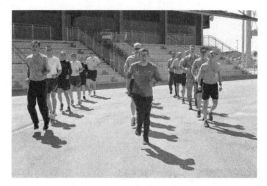

Teaching slow jogging at Air Force Basic Military Training,
Lackland Air Force Base, Texas

outside and moving, it is fun to watch their expressions change. I emphasize soft and springy landings, in addition to the running principles described above—all executed at a slow speed. The endorphins released are evidenced in their smiles.

TAKING IT ALL IN STRIDE

When you overstride and land on your heels you are wasting energy by "braking" just slightly with every step. This reduces the efficiency of forward motion. Overstriding is also associated with more frequent stress injuries, because the forces of impact are absorbed by the bones and joints, which don't store or dissipate

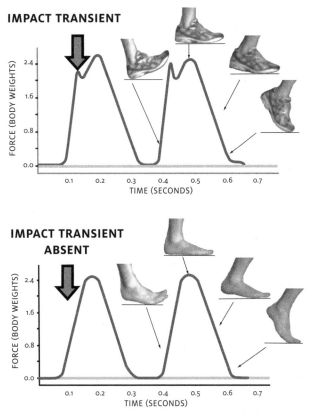

Ground impact forces. Note the impact transient (the tiny, sharp peak of the curve on the top), showing the hard impact caused by rear-foot striking. The figure on the bottom shows a flatter, "softer" impact curve typical of forefoot strikers.

energy well. A slapping sound accompanying each step is one indication of overstriding. Your footfalls should be quiet.

An active, full-foot landing moderates and stores ground impact energy: the falling weight of your body loads the tendons of the foot and ankle, quadriceps, and hips, as if compressing springs that release their energy a moment later—in the next step.

Overstriding also tends to result in too much bounce, or up-and-down motion, which further wastes energy. As you develop your form, notice how your head becomes more stable and quiet, and how your arms move like the drive connectors on a steam locomotive. Visualize your body as the train itself: rolling on rails, powering smoothly and solidly forward, with little side-to-side or up-and-down movement. (Some elite-level runners are a bit of an exception: they have such a long stride that they necessarily rise up and down to some degree.)

WAKE YOUR BOOTY

Throughout, make use of the biggest, most important and tireless muscle in your body—the butt. The gluteus maximus—that's right, the booty—applies more force and stability to the ground than any other muscle when we run, and it is the most efficient for generating forward propulsion. The glutes are packed with fatigue-resistant, slow-twitch type 1 fibers (think "red meat"). When you climb stairs, press a shovel into the ground, or stomp grapes for wine, you are using your glutes. If you learn how to run with your booty, you'll never tire. I've never seen a runner or walker injure that particular muscle.

GAZING AT GAIT

So, what are we looking for when we analyze someone's gait? "Reading" gait is tricky, because imperfections are often subtle. You can see movement, but it is difficult to see the forces that accompany the movement without fancy lab tools, such as force plates. It's also hard to distinguish between what appear to be flaws in someone's form and what may simply be their individual style, their particular strategy for movement, or a peculiarity of their anatomical structure.

Careful, gradual gait retraining should be a key ingredient of the injured runner's rehab menu. For performance runners who aren't injured, however, it may be risky to introduce tweaks to their form, because it can sometimes kick them out of a particular groove they've long become adapted to. They may shift forces to different tissues, increasing vulnerability to injury.

Beginners are different, because imperfections in form and gait tend to be basic and obvious, and are often the cause of injury. It's essential that beginners establish low-impact patterns early on. When looking at the gait of beginning runners, I ask that they start with slow jogging, then progress to a moderate pace. Then I have them alternate between running with and without shoes, to determine how footwear affects gait. (They can readily feel this, too.) By listening, watching, and using a video camera, I try to determine:

- Is the posture tall and the head erect? Is the body squarely suspended under the head?
- When each foot strikes the ground, does the core activate and the midsection stay aligned? Is there a gentle "push" by the glutes when trying to increase speed?

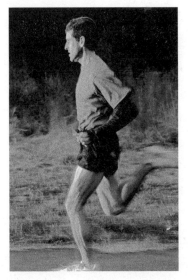

Are the abdominals, legs, and glutes awake and activated?
Think of propelling a skateboard forward.

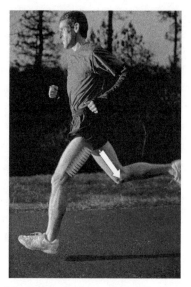

In the forward leg, the hamstring works like a spring
and activates the glutes (arrows), which drive downward,
all in a stretch-contraction reflex, like a bungee cord.

- Are the Achilles tendon, plantar fascia, and calf loaded elastically? There should not be a *thud* with each footstep. If you're on a treadmill, the room shouldn't shake.

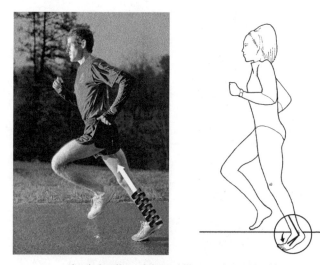

Elastic loading of the Achilles tendon and calf
produces an optimal—quick and powerful—energy return.

- Do the feet naturally pronate (roll inward) in a controlled way, and then supinate (roll outward) to create a stable platform and lever for toe-off?

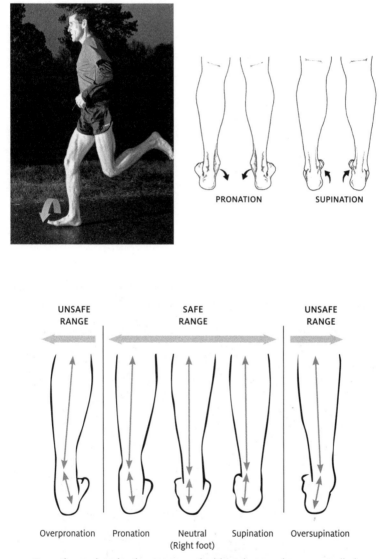

PRONATION   SUPINATION

| UNSAFE RANGE | SAFE RANGE | | | | UNSAFE RANGE |

Overpronation   Pronation   Neutral   Supination   Oversupination
                             (Right foot)

Pronation and supination are normal, although excessive uncontrolled motion can lead to injury. There is a wide range of "normal," however. Overpronating is less common than most people think.

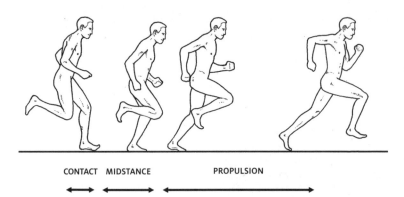

CONTACT MIDSTANCE PROPULSION

Contact, pronation at midstance, supination at propulsion, and toe-off

- When the hip has fully extended, does the knee reflexively spring forward? You shouldn't need to lift the leg with the hip flexors or pull with the hamstring. The action should be relaxed and automatic.

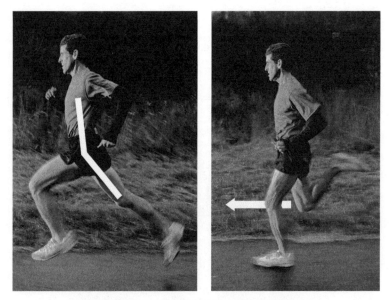

Hip extension loads the springs of the hip flexors.
Then the trailing leg recovers with an elastic, springlike recoil.

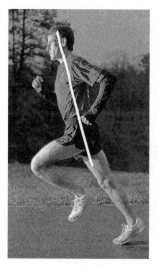
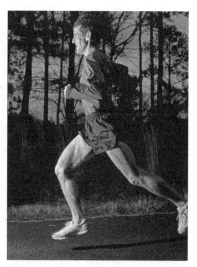

Slight forward lean
at faster running speeds

The point of shoulder rotation is at
the lower thoracic spine. The shoulder
rotates opposite to the hips.

- Is the knee slightly bent on landing, and the lower
  leg perpendicular to the ground? This helps avoid
  overstriding. (See picture on page 81.)
- Is the body upright at a slow jogging pace, but leans
  slightly forward at a faster pace? The runner shouldn't
  bend forward from the waist or hyperextend the back.
- Is the runner's cadence about 180 steps a minute, and is
  there a short ground contact time?
- Are the arms working *for* or *against* the runner? Are the
  elbows bent at 90 degrees or less, and the hands moving
  in a slight circular motion close to the chest? Knuckles
  shouldn't stray far from the sternum, nor cross the center
  line. Is there evidence of rearward pull, as if chopping
  wood, and are the shoulders rotating slightly?
- What is the strategy for increasing speed? Does the
  cadence remain fairly constant, while the stride length
  changes? At faster speeds, the stride angle (see the angle
  of the thighs in full stride, page 90) opens as more force
  is applied to the ground. The ability to easily extend the
  stride indicates good mobility and hip extension.

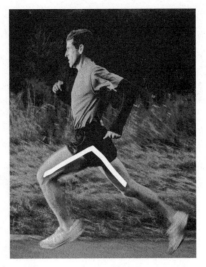

A large stride angle. Note the arms driving back,
as if chopping wood.

- Are the pelvis and hips in positions of strength? At midstance the pelvis should be level, with minimal crossover of the legs. The feet land under the hips, and the pelvis is supported with a strong hip and core.

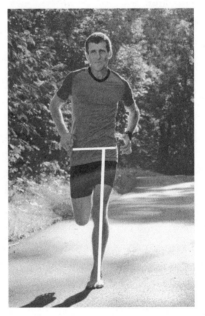

A level pelvis, and minimal leg crossover

AN UNCONVENTIONAL TREADMILL

At my running store in West Virginia, we have been teaching running form with the help of a simple device that has an unusual
ability to fix flaws especially in body position: the TrueForm Runner, a motorless treadmill. The deck of this innovative machine is
slightly bowed—concave from front to back—such that it offers
some resistance as you move the belt.

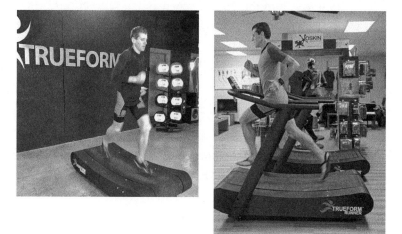

The TrueForm Runner, a runner-powered treadmill

The TrueForm is helpful for doing self-analysis of gait, because
it's impossible to run smoothly and comfortably on it unless you
have good balance, posture, rhythm, glute function, and hip extension. You provide the motive power for the treadmill, and adjustments to your pace and form are entirely up to you. You cannot
overstride, because extending your foot in front and landing on
your heel slows or stops the motion of the belt. Similarly, the concave design demands that you engage the powerful muscles in the
posterior chain, especially the glutes, to keep everything moving.
It's a true "lie detector" of running form.

Adults and kids are invited in to run and play on this treadmill
in our store, and I've enjoyed seeing them relearn their balance
through trial and error (or trial and effort, if you like). Children
get it and adjust almost immediately. They learn unconsciously—
quickly developing the neural pathways needed to initiate and sustain efficient movement.

A varsity runner from the local high school was having knee pain, and I had him hop on the treadmill. I could see that he was tight in the hips (as most runners are), and wasn't fully engaging his glutes. Despite his high level of fitness, he had difficulty moving the belt. He stepped off the treadmill and did exercises to open up his hips (Mountain Climbers, in the drills from the previous chapter) and to activate his glutes (running in place while pulling against a tether, described on pages 94–95.). Then he hopped back on the TrueForm. I gave him some simple cues, and he was off and flying. "A lightbulb switched on," he later said, "and my knee pain has disappeared."

When you don't overstride, and at the same time activate the posterior chain (the glutes and hamstrings), the patellar compressive forces are lessened. The knee can then function as the *hinge* it was meant to be—*not* as a *shock absorber*. This routine won't fix all knee pain, but it often helps in cases of anterior knee pain. Fixing the gait is the first line of treatment—not part-specific rehab. The TrueForm helps runners recognize the motion and the cues that they need to reproduce during their daily training.

AND, RELAX . . .

When making any change to your form—to any routine, really—you should make it incrementally. Your body will adapt, as long as the forces and loads applied do not exceed the natural capacity to recover from some mild, consistent new stresses. Mild to moderate stress ("eustress") with adequate recovery time leads to positive adaptation and strength.

Too many of us are tight and constrained when we run, including in the upper body. The shoulders, arms, and hands should be relaxed. To facilitate this, you can take a few seconds before you run to "shake yourself loose." When you begin running, think about your hands. Instead of a fist, imagine holding potato chips between your fingers. (This is probably the only good use for potato chips.) Try relaxing your lower jaw.

When you practice and train, remember that your feet, legs, and body are doing what they were built for. As children, we ran,

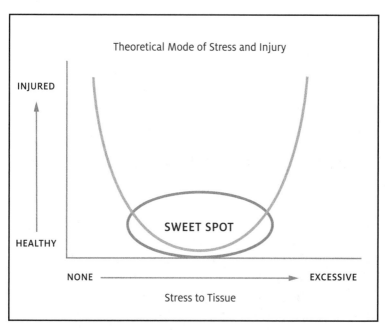

The "sweet spot" represents the area of beneficial eustress.
Greater or lesser levels of stress don't build health or fitness.

jumped, and bounded in our bare feet, as if on springs. We still have much of this near-magical childlike elasticity and bounce. We just need to wake up our natural springs, dial them into a pattern of fluid operation, and enjoy the ride.

DRILLS

Drills for developing efficient, safe running form are easy to perform and generate little harmful impact, if done correctly and progressively. Throughout, keep your balance centered and your position neutral. Pain and injury tend to originate with bad posture.

Study the short list of drills below and try them. They should be performed at least twice a week for progression, then once a week for maintenance, preferably on a day when you aren't fatigued. Warm up with at least ten to fifteen minutes of light running. (I prefer doing drills at the end of runs when I'm warm and loose.) Cut your run a bit short if you need to allocate ten to fifteen minutes to practicing the drills.

Throughout, the goal is to reinforce proper movement patterns and technique, not to build fitness. As the five principles of good running form converge into smooth, efficient movement, these patterns will become your normal default form.

Form = function

- *Jog slowly in your bare feet* on a firm surface. It's safe to take your shoes off and jog tediously slow, even more slowly than a walk. This teaches you impact moderating behavior. Visualize horses trotting out gently to the starting gate at a stakes race. *Tap, tap, tap,* not *thud, thud, thud.* Start with a minute or two.
- To avoid injury, it's important to *reset and maintain your balance* in all planes—front to back, and side to side. Too often, runners sustain injuries that could be prevented by a daily maintenance routine of balancing the body. The simplest balance drill for running is *one-legged running:* run five steps on one leg (with quick on-and-off-the-ground movement), then switch legs and repeat. Slowly build this drill until you can do it for two to three minutes, alternating legs.
- A safe and effective drill for feeling and activating the glutes, and for cadence and foot placement, is to *run*

in place with a tether. Perform this drill on the ground or on a mini-trampoline. With a stretchy tether (such as a mountain bike inner tube) restraining you, you'll see that it doesn't work to use your hamstrings or your hip flexors to lift your legs with each step. Throughout, think about *driving the foot down and back, and popping off the ground* (or mini-trampoline surface) *with your glutes.* Work on your coordination and balance as you do this. Alternatively, turn this into a power drill and try pulling a tire or a sled.

- The *razor scooter* or skateboard is fun, and also excellent practice for foot placement. Powering forward requires extending from the hip while using the glutes. It's not possible to propel a scooter with an overstride, heel-landing pattern.

- Run forward while *skipping rope.* This helps build posture, balance, foot placement, and rhythm, and helps you find your natural cadence. It activates your feet and reduces ground contact time, and makes it difficult to overstride. If skipping rope feels "sticky," be sure to add it to your routine, even if only for a couple of minutes each day.

- View the samples of good and bad running posture shown in the short video clip "1, 2, 3, Run!" (on the videos page of the book's website), and begin your workouts with this drill. Get tall. Run in place with a springy cadence. Then move your face a bit forward. You are off and running!

Watch and learn

The goal of all of these drills is to become "unconsciously competent"—to reach the relaxed, natural state of not having to think about what you are doing. It may be helpful to watch efficient running form in action, as illustrated in "Principles of Natural Running with Dr. Mark Cucuzzella" on the videos page of runforyourlifebook.com. I'm barefoot in this footage to best demonstrate the complex movement of the foot and ankle. Long-distance barefoot running may not be for everyone, but over short distances on a safe surface it will help you learn how your feet and body move without shoes. You'll find that barefoot running is difficult if you have poor form because, quite simply, forceful impact with the ground hurts. You have no choice but to run softly and correctly. Our feet are messengers from the world around us, and they have much to teach. But before we get there, let's build some strength and endurance, which we'll do in the next chapter.

CHAPTER 7

The Engine That Runs Us:
Building Endurance

*You are not training to run an event. What you are training
for is to live a long and productive life and maintain health
optimally. For that there is no question that whatever is
sustainable is the best type of training.*

—DR. TIM NOAKES

MYTH: *High-intensity, push-the-envelope workouts will make
you stronger, and you can forgo low-intensity workouts.*

FACT: *High-intensity training, in isolation, creates a toxic,
acidic environment in your muscles. It inhibits aerobic
development, and will ultimately break you down.*

MYTH: *When you are exercising, sugar is the best fuel to keep
you going.*

FACT: *Fat is a more efficient fuel than sugar; it causes less
physiological stress, and produces greater quantities of useful
energy.*

Now that we're properly "positioned" for running, it's time to
work on the endurance that will lengthen our distances, improve
our times, and restore our health.

A few years ago I got to know a thirty-six-year-old Air Force
musician named Adam Porter. Like many other Airmen, he

trained intensively but minimally for a short period just prior to the annual Air Force fitness test, hoping to regather enough fitness to get a passing grade. But as he "trained," he lost the modest gains he'd made to a combination of burnout, overexertion, and boredom. One year, he failed the test outright, then tried again—and failed again. He had four sons to support, yet was at risk of forfeiting his military career.

I spent a day with him discussing running technique, nutrition, and the concept of maximum aerobic fitness. Mainly, I wanted him to start his training gradually (and well ahead of the test), and to elevate his heart rate to no more than 70 percent of its maximum. Sticking to this plan reduced him to a jog not much speedier than a fast walk. But at the slow pace of 12 minutes and 30 seconds per mile, he was able to work on the principles of natural running form: slowing down, maintaining his balance and gait, not overstriding, bounding, or plodding. Just a smooth, fluid stride.

It took seven months, but Adam shaved four minutes off his mile time. He can now run a mile in 8½ minutes at a heart rate of less than 140 beats per minute. His weight went from 215 pounds to 185.

"My goal is to score in the *90s* on the fitness test," Adam told me, "and to break my 10K personal record of 47:11." By following the endurance methods explained in this chapter, Adam was able to reach his goal. He scored 100 percent on the running portion of the fitness test.

Most all of us can readily do the same thing.

IT ALL STARTED BACK . . .

In the 1960s, a New Zealand running coach named Arthur Lydiard became a national legend when he guided his team to an unprecedented string of five gold medals, two silver medals, and two bronze medals in the Olympics. Lydiard had developed a revolutionary training regimen that—counterintuitively—was based on *slowing down* training speeds for medium and long distances. He exhorted his runners to "train, don't strain" by having them run at a consistent, relaxed, comfortable pace. This technique, and the principles of physiology that Lydiard drew upon, now guides virtually all endurance-building training programs, and it is widely accepted as the surefire means to building a foundation for *health* and *fitness.*

EVERYTHING IS CONNECTED

Let's take a moment to look at the remarkable biology and physiology that make this work.

As we breathe (from the diaphragm, especially), oxygen diffuses from the lungs into the bloodstream, where it attaches to hemoglobin in the blood. The circulatory system (especially where it branches out to the tiniest blood vessels, our 60,000 miles of capillaries) delivers the oxygen-rich hemoglobin to the working muscles to engage in aerobic activity. We're off and running.

If oxygen is a good thing, you'd think that hyperventilating would help boost oxygen delivery and improve performance. Instead, you feel lightheaded when you hyperventilate, because you are blowing off carbon dioxide, too, and a low level of CO_2 in the blood increases the oxygen molecules' affinity for hemoglobin. Breathing more slowly allows CO_2 levels to naturally rise, which expedites offloading of oxygen to the tissues.

We don't live (and run) by oxygen alone. Fuel is needed, too, and is stored in the liver as liver glycogen, in the muscles as muscle glycogen, and to a lesser degree in the blood, as blood glucose. (Our blood contains only a teaspoon of glucose, and this level must be maintained within a narrow range. Thus the blood offers no effective sugar storage, nor a buffer against fluctuations. Think of releasing a constant flow of water from an impoundment, but with no reservoir for storage.)

We also carry with us an abundant supply of fuel as lipids, mainly in the form of triglycerides, the building blocks of fat. Some of this fat energy is stored in the belly and around our internal organs as visceral fat, or *white fat*—the unhealthy kind (that is also difficult to shed). By contrast, fat stored in subcutaneous tissue, or *brown fat,* is metabolically healthy fat. So is *muscular fat,* which is carried in our *intramuscular stores.* The latter two fats are more accessible to us for metabolism and as energy sources than belly fat. Brown fat is abundant with mitochondria.

THE MIGHTY MITOCHONDRIA

The magic happens when the oxygen and fuel converge in the billions of mitochondria—the powerful energy factories within the cells that are stationed around and through our muscle fibers. Each cardiac muscle cell contains about five thousand mitochondria. A biceps muscle has about two hundred. These mitochondria transform potential energy into motion by converting the glycogen and glucose into ATP (adenosine triphosphate, the currency of muscle contraction).

At the same time, through a different process, the triglycerides (building blocks of fat) are mobilized into *free fatty acids* and *glycerol.* This is helped along by lipoprotein lipase (LPL), a hormone-sensitive enzyme, through aerobic processes called oxidative phosphorylation and beta oxidation. These are then converted (in the mitochondria) to the ATP that the muscles demand. Amino acids from protein enter this cycle, too, but to a lesser degree.

Ultimately, how we metabolize our fuel—the efficiency with

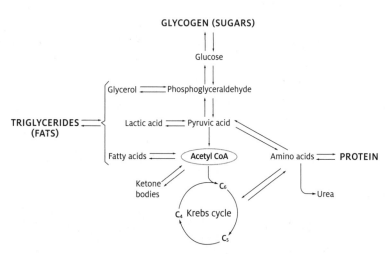

The multiple substrates and fuel pathways of aerobic metabolism, leading to the Krebs cycle and oxidative phosphorylation, to produce ATP. Glycogen and triglycerides are the main fuels that we draw upon for locomotion, but protein can also be broken down into glucose through a process called gluconeogenesis. This isn't the optimal use of proteins, however, as they are needed for other, "higher," nonlocomotive functions in the maintenance of health.

which we convert it into movement and expel waste products—determines how far and fast we run.

THE TWO PRIMARY SYSTEMS OF METABOLISM

For a moment, think of the human body as a car, with the lungs as the air intake; the liver and muscle glycogen as small fuel tanks; our body fat as the large fuel tank; the heart as fuel pump; the mitochondria as spark plugs; and our working muscles and fascia as pistons.

Although visceral (belly) fat may form the largest fuel tank, it suffers from an annoying problem: its prodigious reserves of energy are mostly locked up, and aren't readily accessible for use by our muscles. This is why belly fat, unfortunately, is so difficult to shed.

A more apt comparison is to a *hybrid* vehicle, because the fuel in our bodies is burned via two converging metabolic pathways—sugar burning and fat burning. These two metabolic systems work together, not unlike the paired-up combo of a gasoline engine and an electric motor. Let's take a look at how they combine forces to make the human body the most efficient rig on the road:

The sugar-burning "gasoline" system (mix of anaerobic and high-end aerobic)

When you sprint or make an explosive, momentary effort, you are burning glucose, a quickly metabolized, high-octane sugar. The muscles almost instantly convert glucose to ATP and deliver short bursts of high energy. This is comparable to stomping on the gas and using the hybrid car's gasoline engine exclusively—which can be handy for powering quickly up a steep, short hill to pass a truck.

This capability has been useful to us throughout our evolution (think fight or flight), but only for about one minute at a stretch. There's simply insufficient lead time to get a sustained dose of oxygen into the muscles for this instantaneous, on-demand form of energy. And this mostly anaerobic system (it occurs in the absence of oxygen) is limited by the toxic accumulation of acidic by-products—the equivalent of excessive, dark exhaust, in the car analogy. Hard sustained exercise uses the high end of the aerobic system and depletes the sugar/gas quickly and is also "exhaust" heavy.

The fat-burning "electric" system (pure aerobic)

To increase endurance and efficiency, on the other hand, we need to transition out of the sugar-burning "gas guzzling" mode, and switch to the more efficient, fat-burning "electric" system. It's a cherished myth that if you are exercising at your peak efficiency, sugar is the best fuel to keep you going. In fact, fat is a far more useful energy source, because it offers much more ATP per molecule than sugar does. The metabolic by-products ("exhaust") from burning fat are cleaner, too, resulting in less harmful inflammation. (Ketone bodies are one product of aerobic-fat metabolism, and have been described as a "super-fuel"—a clean source of energy that can be used directly by the brain and muscle.) As long as you're burning fat, you'll pass the smog test.

When driving a hybrid car, you often can't detect the subtle mixing of gas and electricity. Similarly, your exercising body constantly draws upon a changing mix of fat and sugar. But any vigorous effort lasting more than an hour is best performed in "electric"— aerobic, sustainable, comfortable, fat-burning—mode. When running aerobically on fat, we become resistant to breakdown and can run all day on a minimum of added fuel.

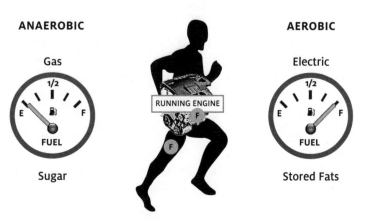

A full battery wins the long-distance race.

THE TRAINING ZONES

When training, racing, or simply exerting at any activity, it is help-ful to have an idea of the metabolic "training zone" that your body is operating in. These zones, and the thresholds that demarcate them, aren't precise. But as you dial in awareness of your exertion level, you'll be better able to gauge your fuel consumption and how long you can endure at a given level of effort.

- The *aerobic zone* is the lowest-level training range, in which you are functioning almost entirely aerobically, burning fat. The upper part of this zone corresponds to your maximum aerobic heart rate, and your ventilatory (or aerobic) threshold. Building health and endurance, and density of mitochondria, happens primarily in this zone. Paradoxically, strong aerobic training pushes up your anaerobic threshold (AT, see page 104), too, because a well-developed aerobic system is packed with functioning mitochondria and better buffers acidity.
- The *aerobic threshold* (AeT), or ventilatory threshold (VT), is the mostly imperceptible line dividing the pure aerobic zone (in which you are burning primarily fat for energy) and the glucose-burning zone (in which you are burning the more accessible but far less abundant glycogen and glucose). When you are near this threshold, your exertion is aerobic, with minimal or no anaerobic contribution because you are still using your near-bottomless tank of fat. Your daily training goal is to stay near this threshold while remaining in the aerobic zone. You can use this simple feedback tool: when your respiratory rate picks up, or when you can no longer breathe through your nose, dial down your exertion a notch. (You'll see this on a group run, for instance, when everyone is relaxed and conversational, then someone picks up the pace and conversation ceases.) Consistently creeping above the AeT/VT can lead to increased fatigue, poor recovery, and overall adrenal stress.
- Between the AeT/VT and anaerobic threshold is the

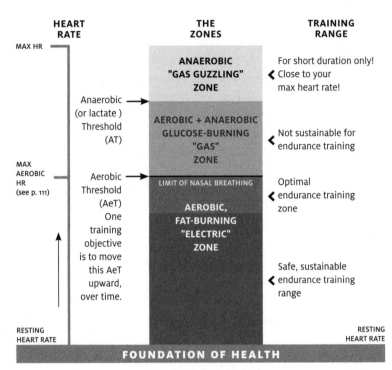

see p. 111

The Training Zones

glucose-burning zone, where both aerobic and anaerobic metabolisms are operational. The rate of exertion remains tolerable, which means that acidity is buffered and doesn't accumulate in the system. Racing and periodic workouts in this zone can work for those who are in excellent aerobic health. Many people routinely train in this zone, yet doing so for extended periods is not compatible with building health and endurance.

• At the top, at the highest level of exertion, are the *anaerobic threshold* and the *anaerobic zone.* When the level of exertion surpasses the anaerobic threshold (AT, also known as the lactate threshold), the body cannot buffer the acidity, and acid begins to accumulate in the muscles. When you're out of shape, you may reach this threshold quickly, even during a slow jog. The AT of elite athletes, by comparison, is close to their maximum level of exertion, meaning that they can operate at a high level of performance and still remain just *below* their

AT. Training *above* the AT is difficult and stressful. (For performance athletes, training in the anaerobic zone can be useful at times, but the small increment of fitness they gain can come at the cost of aerobic development and risk of overtraining and injury.)

In summary, training constantly in the upper zones—above the AeT/VT—can be harmful. We have recently become aware that years of high-intensity training increase the risk of atrial fibrillation, right heart failure, and myocardial fibrosis. Humans, in order to survive, were designed to move efficiently and comfortably over long distances, with occasional bursts of speed. We *weren't* designed to run ten hard miles every day at an anaerobic threshold pace.

SO, WHAT DOES THIS MEAN FOR HOW WE EXERCISE?

As you exercise and train, you can learn to sense which zone you are in and which threshold you might be near. When the blood glucose and muscle glycogen level—the gas tank—is depleted, we crash, or "bonk," as runners say. The body signals the brain (which strives to maintain a constant blood sugar level) to tell the runner to slow down, stop, or take in nourishment immediately.

Many of us run too hard, yet we get away with it by trying to replenish our easily accessed but quickly depleted glycogen gas tanks in the liver and the muscles. For the fatigued or bonked runner, however, topping off the tank with *more* sugar, followed by high levels of effort, only repeats the cycle of eating, exertion, and exhaustion. By analogy, it's better to feed a hot fire by throwing on a log (fat) than by constantly feeding it paper or twigs (sugar).

Months and years of aerobic training and proper diet can make you a "better butter burner"—as in fat burner. One common measure of cardiorespiratory fitness (especially endurance) is an individual's maximum rate of oxygen consumption, or VO_2 max, which can be measured during exercise of increasing intensity. What's interesting is that two people with the same measured VO_2 max—two runners with nominally the same level of maximum endurance—can exhibit, in running lab tests, a marked difference in their abilities to burn sugars or to burn fats. "Fat adapted" athletes can run close to their AT while still burning fat while sugar-dependent athletes switch to sugar at low intensities. In endurance training sessions or long events especially, those who have "trained" their enzymes and metabolism to burn long-lasting fat calories will pull away from those whose bodies have become dependent on stored and ingested sugar. I encourage you to visit runforyourlifebook.com for my discussion about this, "Burn Fat for Health and Performance: Better Butter Burner," where I share the results of my 2017 test.

POWER CENTERS AND PATHWAYS

To successfully build our endurance engine (and boost overall health), we need to increase the density of the mitochondria and capillaries in our muscles. This is done through consistent, sustained exercise of light to moderate intensity, and efficient delivery of oxygen to the muscles.

Our bodies can burn glucose and glycogen for only a short period. But most of us, even if our body profile appears lean, have a functionally limitless reserve of fat. We can tap into fat metabolism by slowing down and training within the pure aerobic zone, while maintaining a diet full of healthy fats.

The burning of fat greatly boosts the efficiency of our mitochondrial machinery. Accessing fat provides the environment for building more mitochondrial power centers and more capillary pathways, meaning that even *more* fat can be metabolized for training runs and races—and for the military's 1.5-mile fitness test.

The physiology and chemistry is complex, but the practical implications for us are straightforward: the more capillaries and mitochondria we have, the more ATP they produce and the stronger and faster the muscles contract without fatiguing. When you create the demand for long-term performance, the body responds by creating the machinery. This is the hybrid's electric engine: never empty and always recharging, as long as you eat healthy fats and maintain a comfortable pace. In the car analogy, you are morphing from a Charger to a Prius, and ultimately to a Tesla, as your electric engine grows.

RED / AEROBIC MUSCLE

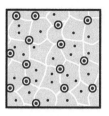
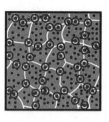

⊙ Capillaries
• Mitochondria

No Endurance Training   After Endurance Training

The long-term effect of comfortable endurance training:
more energy-delivering capillaries and mitochondria expand
and perfuse into the muscles.

Running coach Arthur Lydiard was aware of this. His method of training the best middle- and long-distance runners began with months—even years—of aerobic training. His runners launched the foundational part of their training regimen with easy, aerobic runs—mostly in the comfortable, fat-burning aerobic zone. His 800-meter specialists trained by going on twenty-two-mile runs, and they racked up a hundred miles a week. The reason was simple: he wanted his runners to build a massive and resilient aerobic system. As competitive events approached, he turned up the intensity, by gradual and measured increments, until the runners were pushing their maximum capacity.

For most athletes, six weeks of high-intensity training before an event seems to be the maximum tolerated training period before their level of performance peaks and then may even start to decline as the runner begins to overreach and overtrain. (See chapter 11 on recovery to better understand the important role that *rest* plays in building strength and endurance.) Muscoloskeletal injury is also associated with high-intensity training over extended periods.

I'm not suggesting that you run twenty-two miles at a pop, or a hundred miles a week, but these principles still apply to almost all modern training programs. A carefully gauged progression works to optimize the body's daily eustress—the *optimum* dose of physiological stress that builds health and imparts a feeling of fulfillment. At this moderate level of stress, *neovascularization* and *biogenesis* occur in the heart, too, whereby areas of the heart grow new blood vessels and the cells remodel, and more mitochondria and capillaries are formed. This results in a richer network for oxygen and nutrient delivery.

In the year 2000, I began to experiment with pure aerobic training speeds, and as I slowed down, the faster I got—at the same level of easy effort. I began by running ten-minute miles at a heart rate of 150. Six months later, I was running six-minute miles at the same heart rate. That fall, I entered the thirty-thousand-runner Marine Corps Marathon, and finished third, without having done any hard running or speed work.

At the finish line, I was surprised by an unusual sensation, compared with previous races: I felt that I could turn around and do it again. It's common for runners to feel, after training in the aerobic zone for a few weeks, that they have more energy *after* their workout than when they began. Try it yourself.

In the early 1960s, Lydiard introduced "jogging" to New Zealanders, and eventually to the world. He also developed the first cardiac rehabilitation program that included jogging as part of its therapy. He knew that *relaxed movement* was the secret to recovery from heart disease, and he encouraged cardiac patients to build up to thirty minutes of jogging a day (at a conversational pace), over a period of several weeks to months. At that time, by contrast, the U.S. medical establishment was focused on *resting* the body. Since then, we have learned that bed rest, especially, is very damaging to the heart, and we have adopted Lydiard's principles. The thirty-minute a day jogging goal for cardiac rehab is now the foundation of the *Physical Activity Guidelines for Americans*.

In my medical practice, too, I encourage my heart disease patients to slowly ramp up to a jogging pace. Following a heart attack, the heart loses some of its contractility and efficiency. But aerobic training boosts the capacity of the body's muscles by up to 400 percent, which means that the heart needs to work less for any given activity.

Take the case of local runner Mike Foster, a young father of three. At age thirty-eight, Mike was living a healthy, athletic life. He didn't smoke, drank little alcohol, and ate healthfully, but he did have a family history of heart problems. In January 2014 he played a game of basketball and felt some pain in his chest (which he assumed was from an elbow in the ribs) and shortness of breath (which he thought was from being winded, following a two-week vacation).

Mike had suffered a heart attack. He promptly underwent quintuple bypass surgery. Afterward, he committed himself to rehab, and set his sights on entering the Freedom's Run 5K in October of the same year—and he completed it. One year later, following twelve more months of low-intensity training, he broke the tape of the Freedom's Run marathon. His kids were waiting and cheering at the finish line.

By focusing on comfortable training and overall health, Mike no longer has markers of progressive heart disease. He—and increasingly others—have shown that whole body conditioning may be the best form of cardiac rehab.

SLOW AND STEADY WINS THE RACE . . .

Many believe that high-intensity, push-the-envelope workouts make you stronger and fitter than low-intensity workouts. This may work temporarily, but can create a toxic, acidic environment in the muscles, inhibiting the aerobic development that we seek.

Less acute, but just as damaging in the long term, is falling into the "black hole" of training. This comes from consistently training above your aerobic threshold, and not allowing sufficient time for

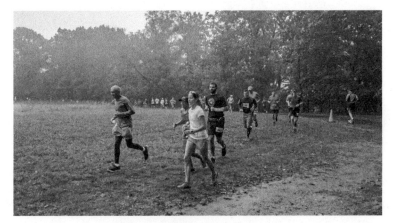

Slow and steady wins the race.

recovery. Many of us do this, and wonder why our performance declines. It distresses me to see people destroying themselves in brutal, intense daily workouts in the name of athletic excellence (or to "make up for lost time"). We need to slow down in order to speed up, and we need to run with joy. As the minimalist running tribe leader and friend Barefoot Ted says, "Don't practice pain. Practice pleasure."

There's no hurry. We are training for the rest of our healthy lives.

DRILLS

To determine the best, sustainable level of exertion for building the aerobic ("electric"), fat-burning engine, it's best to have a trainer or master teacher. But a heart rate monitor can work, plus some simple measurements and record keeping. Once you reach a fitness plateau, you shouldn't even need these.

1. Determine your maximum aerobic heart rate

There are several methods for finding your maximum aerobic heart rate (MAHR)—the sustained rate that will best build your endurance engine. This heart rate (or range, within a few beats per minute) is most easily and safely determined by using the "180 Formula," developed by Dr. Phil Maffetone in 1982. Despite some differences, other methods for calculating this work fine—most of the time. The Karvonen formula and the Friel method, based on lactate threshold, work well, but deriving MAHR from them is more complicated.

Elite athletes Mark Allen and Mike Pigg, among many others, have successfully used the 180 Formula for building a solid foundation for health and world-class performance, and for extending their race careers. I'm confident that you'll discover what we have: although your heart rate remains in check over the weeks and months of training, your endurance, your feeling of well-being, and your speed will improve.

The 180 Formula
Subtract your age from 180 (180 – age). This gives you a baseline beats per minute (bpm).

Then modify this number by selecting adjustments that match your health profile:

- If you have a major illness (heart disease, high blood pressure, etc.), are in recovery from an operation or hospital stay, or are taking medication, subtract an additional 10 bpm.
- If you have never exercised, have been training

inconsistently, have not recently progressed in training or competition, are injured, or get more than two colds or bouts of flu per year or have allergies (or are subject to a combination of these), subtract an additional 5 bpm.
- If you've been exercising regularly (at least four times weekly) for up to two years without any of the problems listed above, keep the number at 180 minus age.
- If you have been competing for more than two years without any of the problems listed above, and have improved in competition without injury, add 5 bpm.

For example, if you are thirty years old and have not been training consistently, then your MAHR would be:

$$180 - 30 = 150, \text{ then } 150 - 5 = \textbf{145 bpm}$$

In my case, I am fifty-one years old and work out at least four times per week, and I've been healthy, so I add 5 bpm to the raw number of 180 minus my age. I end up with a MAHR of **134 bpm**.

Whatever figure results from this calculation, this *maximum aerobic heart rate* generally falls within the range recommended by exercise physiologists as a safe aerobic training heart rate: 60 to 80 percent of one's *maximum heart rate*—the highest rate that your heart should normally reach during extended physical exertion. The 180 Formula is slightly conservative, and therefore especially good if you are new to running, are recovering from an injury, or don't feel sufficiently fit to take on the high-intensity run.

A choice few who are very accomplished at fat burning can be a bit more liberal—with caution—and work out at a maximum aerobic heart rate of 200 minus their age.

And you may find that getting a test of your VO_2 is a very useful tool. By measuring respiratory gases in a physiology lab, it's possible to determine whether you are running in the aerobic zone. The VO_2 max figure that results from this test will give you an idea of your overall aerobic ability. But VO_2 levels at less-than-maximum effort may be even more useful as an indicator of whether you are burning fat or sugar. (As glucose metabolism increases, you produce more CO_2, which signals that you are leaving the fat-burning aerobic training zone and entering the anaerobic zone.) A local exercise physiologist may be able to test your VO_2, or a university sports science department may offer the test for free.

2. Measure your progress—with one simple assignment

Assuming you are committed to improving your overall aerobic fitness, then how do you track your progress? For that matter, how can you be certain that you are improving at all? The feeling that you are becoming healthier and aerobically fit is often subjective, especially for those who haven't been exercising regularly. But once you know your maximum aerobic heart rate, a simple way to measure progress is to apply what's called the *maximal aerobic function* test:

- Find a two- to three-mile route, preferably flat.
- As you run (or walk) the route, stay within your optimal aerobic training zone (don't exceed the MAHR that you calculated above). Record your time over the route.
- Do most or all of your running in this aerobic zone for several weeks—regardless of the terrain or the distances or the places you run; throughout, work on form, relaxation, breathing, and rhythm (as you read about in chapter 6), while staying at or below your MAHR. Running efficiency is all about creating mechanical and metabolic advantage.
- Repeat the test every couple of weeks, timing your original route under similar conditions each time. (Heat will cause the heart rate to drift up, and wind will affect your speed.)
- Record your time. This is your "aerobic speed," and you will see it gradually progress—just as it did for Adam Porter (at the beginning of the chapter). Some of your improvement will result from the increased efficiency of your metabolism, and some from improvements in form and biomechanics.

With experience, you should be able to remain in your aerobic training zone simply by sensing your level of effort, without a heart rate monitor. Feel the rhythm of your breathing and your level of exertion, pay attention to your feelings, set mental reference points, and learn the language of your physiology. Develop your own system of biofeedback. One reliable way to do this is to limit yourself to breathing through your nose. If you can maintain a genuine smile, too, you will feel as if you can run forever.

Once your times on the two- to three-mile course are no longer improving—typically after several months, and sometimes years— you have fully built your aerobic endurance engine! You will notice that you are faster than ever before, yet running at a level of exertion that is as easy and comfortable as the day you began.

In some instances, it may be necessary for your heart rate to drift above your MAHR:

- At the end of a long training session, especially in warm weather, as long as you are feeling comfortable and can carry on a conversation. Your heart rate naturally kicks up to help cool you.
- During short sprints and drills (of around ten seconds), which I do almost daily. My heart rate climbs for a few seconds, then I allow it to settle down before the next short sprint.
- As a race approaches, I'll pick up my pace four to six weeks before the event maybe once or twice a week. (See chapter 12, on racing.)

It's probably not helpful to train with a group that runs at a pace that will take you above your own MAHR, at least not every day. On a group run, your heart rate will naturally climb as the pace quickens. When you crest a hill or when the pace settles, focus on relaxing and recovering.

CHAPTER 8

Move More and "Exercise" Less

Lack of activity destroys the good condition of every human being, while movement and methodical physical exercise save it and preserve it.

—PLATO

Don't exercise beyond the limit of your brain's ability to control a movement properly.

—DAVID WEINSTOCK, physical therapist and author

MYTH: *You should stretch thoroughly before a workout.*

FACT: *This is not advised. Simply jog gently to melt the "fuzz" in the fascia; swing the arms and skip a little to open up the range of motion.*

In this chapter, I'm going to suggest that you don't need to "exercise" at all.

Since the invention of the yardstick and the stopwatch, we have been *quantifying* movement. The government releases important-sounding guidelines on the minimum number of minutes of daily exercise. People rush to their gyms and dutifully perform their routines, while GPS devices track their movements and social media hails their hero workouts.

Most of us who become committed to a workout regimen subscribe to the popular acronym FIT—*frequency, intensity,* and *time*. But often our exercise is *too* vigorous, at the same time that it doesn't address the damage caused by parking ourselves in a chair for the rest of the day. Even if we run for 30 minutes, what about the 930 other minutes of daily nonsleep time?

Modern humans share with zoo animals the diseases of captivity. We exercise to compensate for restricted habitat and range. And we regard exercise as we do nutritional supplements. Just as supplements shouldn't be the foundation of our diet, exercise routines shouldn't form the bulk of our daily movement.

INVISIBLE TRAINING

We have sidelined movement from our daily routines. For physical health alone, if you simply move through a wide range of motions throughout the day, "exercise" becomes redundant. Our bodies are meant to be used, and movement is what they are adapted for. *Exercise* is great. But the only genuine, healthful, and sustainable reason to exercise is because you love it.

In medical school, I was taught anatomy and the configuration of the human body—a *static* human body. And as a doctor in the clinic, I "examined" patients who were sitting passively on a table, without assessing their movement. Only later would I begin to understand the fluid mechanics and marvelous interconnectedness of a body in motion.

When I'm asked, "What is the best position or movement?" I respond by saying, "Your *next* one." If you have remained in any single position for more than twenty minutes, change it up. As you do, expand the ways you reposition your tissues and load your joints. Each time you stress and move new areas, local blood circulation increases. Mix up the ways in which you interact with the environment—just as our ancestors did constantly.

Running alone isn't enough to get you to a state of excellent health. In addition to running, we need to engage in a *variety* of activities and movements. Walking, lifting objects (properly), gardening, squatting, crawling, climbing stairs—all of these "supplemental movements" should be done briskly and with graceful ease, and at frequent intervals throughout the day. In other words, apply the level of attention that you bring to your running form to *all* of your movements, and regard yourself as in a constant state of "invisible training."

The "isolation training" that many people do in gyms often consists of programs for narrow, specific purposes, and isn't always healthful. Instead, by teaching the body to link its movements and become one machine, not a Frankenstein-like assemblage of parts, you will be far more suited to many functional and athletic tasks.

A STANDING ORDER

For a moment, let's tag back to the most damaging habit that we've subjected our bodies to: chronic sitting. As we discussed in chapter 2, sitting is associated with a number of physical problems and chronic ailments, and prolonged sitting increases the likelihood of an earlier death. Consider plane flights: typically, we drive (in a sitting position) to the airport, cram ourselves into an airplane's economy seat, then again drive (while sitting) to our destination, in order to sit at a meeting or sit around with friends. It surprises me to see people without roller bags in airport terminals congregate at the base of the escalators, when the wonderful opportunity of stairs—which are generally faster—waits nearby, unused. We should all be taking every opportunity to *move*.

After hours in a chair, our muscles and fascia essentially reprogram themselves, misaligning our entire kinetic chain. Hips tighten, hip flexors shorten, and the gluteus maximus gets "remodeled," such that we lose the optimal tension, spring, and range of motion that is needed for efficient walking and running.

In what some researchers have termed the "active couch potato" phenomenon, the negative effects of prolonged sitting may cancel out the gains accrued from exercise, even when the exercise includes training for a marathon or half marathon. (Emerging research that traces the roles of inflammatory- and fat-regulating enzymes, such as LPL1, also supports this.) Runners and others who train vigorously may be at higher risk: they tend to be professionals, confined to long hours at a desk or in a car. They may rationalize, however subconsciously—but incorrectly—that their extraordinary exercise efforts more than compensate for any risks from a mostly sedentary life.

Prolonged muscular *in*activity, as experienced on long plane rides, can also place someone at risk of deep vein thrombosis (DVT), or blood clots. A flight from New York to Germany entails less sitting than an eight-hour workday at a desk. We may need to start seriously examining the health effects of our ubiquitous sedentary daily lives.

A stand-up desk is a partial antidote to sitting, and I have used one for over ten years. The desk holds my laptop, phone, and papers, and I keep a stool beside it to elevate a foot to change position while I read and type. At home, I rarely sit in chairs, and take every opportunity to sit on the floor and change up my position, as if in a yoga class. We can all do this. Visualize yourself as an ancestral human—unassisted and unconstrained by chairs and tables—versus the modern zoo human.

THE SPICE OF LIFE

Our neuromuscular systems are adaptive and trainable. They enable us to react to, temper, dissipate, redirect, and stabilize large forces. Nerves control muscles (what's meant by "neuromuscular"), and the more we practice and build proprioception and balance, the more neuromuscular control occurs locally—reflexively, automatically—without the intermediate step of engaging the thinking brain.

Fascia plays a role with this (see chapter 5), because it relays signals about when to tighten, loosen, or stabilize, without us needing to cogitate on it. Proprioceptors and mechanoreceptors in our feet and throughout the body sense load, pressure, and blood flow. To some degree, all of this movement and countermovement trickles down to individual cells, and may even affect which genes get turned on and off. Gene expression, we're learning, is a product of what we *do,* not just who we *are.*

When you're walking or running, proprioceptive mechanoreceptors, which generally sit at the nerve endings, send signals to the cells of the muscles in the feet and legs. The cells (which are mostly water) behave like a sponge, and are refreshed by constant filling and squeezing, in just the right amounts. Disuse of the mechanoreceptors (as occurs in prolonged bed confinement) can result in a pressure sore or bedsore. Fluid accumulates in the ankles. The sponge is wrung out or overfilled, and isn't refilling properly. Simply changing up one's position helps move lymph and fluids and blood through the tissues.

YOU GOT TO MOVE IT . . . MOVE IT!

So, if you've been on the couch or at a desk for years and want to expand your range of motion, where do you begin? *Just move, and you will improve.* Bend. Compress. Twist. Pull. Push. Lift. Squat throughout the day, whenever you can. I squat to rub my dog's belly—it's as good for me as it is for her. One hundred squat-jumps in the gym aren't required.

Undertake all of this movement within a safe range of motion. Remember that the body adapts gradually. Never make a sudden or outsized change to your routine or movement patterns (or to your footwear).

The perfect, most accessible movement is walking. It helps us in every way—mechanically, metabolically, psychologically. If you walk outside, all of your senses are stimulated. I am one of few physicians who still does traditional walking rounds: I walk from room to room visiting patients, instead of "rounding" at a circular table with laptops. ("Rounds" originated at the original Johns Hopkins Hospital, where the halls of the ward were configured in a large circle.)

Physical therapist Gary Gray coined a term for the motor control that we need in order to prevent injury and excel in sports: *mostability,* a blending of *mobility* and *stability.* It describes the ability to take advantage of just the right motion, at just the right time, at just the right speed, in just the right plane, and in just the right direction. The objective is to elongate the muscles and move the joints through their full range of motion, while using skillful motor control to manage the forces that are generated.

By contrast, *instability* can be referred to as any degree of mobility that isn't fully controlled.

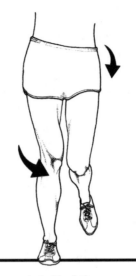

Core instability, exacerbated by fatigue, causes the right knee
to dive in and left hip to drop, leading to decreased motor control
and efficiency—like a tired spring.

TO STRETCH OR NOT TO STRETCH?
THAT IS THE QUESTION.

There's been a lot of discussion about whether one should stretch
before running. The current consensus is that it's not necessary,
and may even be counterproductive.

Some of the confusion arises because stretching can refer to a
variety of routines and movements. In *static stretching,* a specific
position is held for ten or more seconds, as in many types of yoga,
and can be harmful if done *prior* to running. In *active isolated
stretching,* on the other hand, a muscle is contracted and held only
for a moment—at most a few seconds—and then is lengthened.
Repeated several times, this kind of stretching can release neuro-
logic inhibition in the muscles and fascia. (This inhibition, which
may feel like tightness, can indicate that your nervous system is
preventing a joint from moving fully—and may be protecting it
from injury.)

Active isolated stretching can open you up to a wider range of
motion, though it may help only modestly. The goal is to loosen,
not stretch, and the best way to do this is to simply run at an easy,
relaxed pace. At the start of a run, swing the arms and skip a little

LENGTH-TENSION RELATIONSHIP

Overly flexed joints have too much overlap between actin (thin line) and myosin (thick line), making it tough to further shorten the muscle for rapid energy production.

A mild amount of flex in a joint allows the muscles to shorten slightly and optimizes the amount of overlap between fibers for rapid force production.

Too much straightening of the joint lengthens the individual fibers and makes it harder to rapidly shorten the muscle.

to open up the range of motion, then start out jogging slowly to melt the "fuzz" in the fascia. As your body warms up, your mobility and range of motion will expand naturally. Add a few skips, lunges, and even a few short pickups (ten-second sprints), in which you lengthen your stride and test your full range of motion. This is *dynamic stretching*—and is done mostly when you're warmed up.

Indeed, simply keeping your body limber, supple, and active throughout the day is more important than a dedicated program of stretching, or a rigorous menu of positions, yoga poses, and movements. Especially now that we are learning of the increased risk of mortality—early death—from the benign-sounding activity known as *chronic sitting*, we should pay special attention to daily movement.

Remember the tensegrity principle. The body wants to remain in a balanced state between tension and compression. Thus stretching needs to be viewed in the context of *what,* exactly, needs stretching.

Commonly, I see tightness in the anterior hips, or hip flexors. Think of your pelvis and femur secured into a "comma" position, caused by shortened hip flexors that accompany long periods of sitting. (Your frame should be erect, with a flat, neutral pelvis when you stand upright, as in the illustration that follows.) Now combine that comma position with a tight and sore upper hamstring. One might think that stretching the hamstring is a priority,

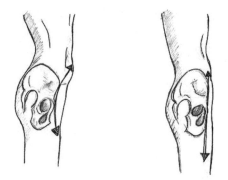

The "comma," or tilted pelvis, at left, is an artifact
of prolonged sitting—compared to a flat, neutral pelvis, at right.

but this will only exaggerate the curve in the "comma" and result in *more* imbalance and compensation.

Ron Clarke, who set seventeen world records, said that he never stretched before running. Yet to watch Ron run was to watch stretching in action. He ran with perfect balance and a full range of motion. You can see (below) that his stride angle (the angle of separation between his thighs) is greater than 90 degrees.

Ron retired from distance running in his prime, at age thirty-three. Meb Keflezighi qualified for the Olympics for the fourth time at age forty. Like Ron, Meb didn't do stretching and mobility work when he was younger. Now, however, he does an extensive series of drills similar to the ones I prescribe, in order to maintain

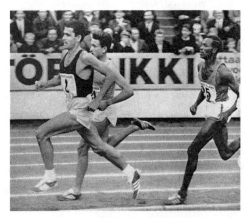

Ron Clarke (#2) in full flight

balance and range of motion. He does them all in a dynamic and relaxed way, never pulling hard on his muscles.

Similarly, you don't want to take your exercise into the exhaustion zone, as your muscles will tighten up on you. I want the final mile of every run to be the most fluid and relaxed of all, with the fullest motion and longest stride. This applies to walking, too. No need for long post-workout stretching sessions. You just stretched, while in motion.

It's simple: after you have worked out comfortably—avoiding exhaustion and cooling down slowly—you are set up for optimal recovery. No need to do anything more. But remember: if you return to the chair immediately after a workout, you'll sabotage the range of motion that just nourished your body. Your muscles and joints and fascia will cool down and "set" in that sitting position, and you'll have to start over the next day. This is similar to spending good time and money on massage or deep tissue work to alleviate positional pain and tightness—then immediately resuming the damaging posture that necessitated the treatment. I witness this daily.

MINIMALIST GOLF? (NO, NOT MINIATURE GOLF.)

Many runners are also golfers, and golf qualifies as a type of full body movement—when done "old school." One of my mentors, Dr. Phil Maffetone, wrote a book called *The Healthy Golfer,* which doesn't prescribe the best grip for your club nor demonstrate the correct swing plane. Instead, it shows you how to lower your score by becoming the healthy, flexible, focused, and relaxed person that the sport demands. As with running, a good golf game requires listening to and caring for your body. Maffetone starts by encouraging golfers to wear shoes with flat, flexible, spikeless soles, and to go barefoot during the day and eat the right foods.

Part of my early aerobic base for running was built on golf. During the summers, beginning at age eleven, I walked eighteen (or more) holes of golf each day with my brothers at our local course. Our golf shoes were Keds and Converse sneakers, and the bag I carried weighed almost as much as I did. We couldn't afford to lose golf balls, and routinely climbed across rocky terrain and forded creeks to retrieve them. We never took lessons, and played with blade clubs—old wooden and steel clubs with tiny sweet spots. As a result, we developed natural swings. Now golfers rely on over-sized titanium clubs like the Big Bertha driver, and often don't get the full feel of the ball and club.

My wife, Roberta, and I continue to play, and when in Colorado we found a little-known course called Perry Park that is tucked into the red rocks of Colorado. Walking is encouraged there, and we were allowed to bring our dog. Eighteen holes took us three hours, and we finished more refreshed than when we set out. The grounds crew even allowed us to go on morning runs.

Later, we experienced golf at its purest on a trip to Ireland. The terrain was impassable for a cart, and the elderly caddies were the healthiest and strongest seniors I have met. Most courses in the United States now require that golfers ride carts. Walking is prohibited! I tried a cart once, and found that in addition to feeling lethargic, I couldn't concentrate on my form or the game. I'm a minimalist golfer, and love it that way. I carry six clubs, each more than twenty-five years old, and still play a decent game. My favorite "golf" shoes are FiveFingers or running sandals. Our local course in West Virginia still encourages walking, and they allow me to run there during the early morning hours, too.

My father-in-law is in his nineties, and he walks the course (with four clubs). A few years ago, a group of young players in carts came upon him.

"How old are you?" one young man asked.

"Ninety," he replied.

"Wow. I hope I can still get out on the course when I'm ninety," the young man said.

"Then get out of the cart," my father-in-law responded.

Golf can be a source of health and fitness for anyone. But the modern version of it—the electric carts, stiff shoes with spikes, and heavy bags with too many clubs—robs golfers of the experience of mastering the game from the ground up. In golf, as in running, the feet and their connection to the earth greatly affect what happens to the rest of the body, and how you perform.

DRILLS

The drills here are all about expanding mobility and range of motion. Each of these movements should leave you feeling refreshed and ready to go again the next day, not sore and unable to move. The *quality* of your movement is more important than how much weight you lift or how fast you perform a task or a drill. Three years from now, no one will care how well you performed in today's workout, but injuring yourself is an event you'll likely remember.

Whether you are a competitor or exercising for fun and fitness, *train the pattern, not the part.* The brain and nervous system do not recognize individual muscles; they recognize patterns of movement.

Exercise snacks between meals

"Exercise snacks" can help break up the day and get the blood flowing. I spend much of my hospital workday walking. Between patients, I often stretch and do gentle lunges and trunk twists. If you work in an office, exercise snacks such as these will keep you healthy and flexible. You can stand while chatting with a colleague or student, and phone conversations offer more opportunities to stretch and move.

When working from home, interrupt your day by going outside and completing chores, especially those that demand some physical effort. When you return to your desk (preferably a stand-up variety), you are physically and mentally refreshed, and noticeably more productive.

In the following drills, we are going to work on *movements, not muscles,* and progress from very simple to more complex. You need not do all of these, but they can populate the menu that you select from, depending on the level of challenge you desire, and how it fits in your day.

Let's start with some mobility assessments.

Ankle mobility assessment
Place your right foot forward with your toes about four inches from a wall. With heels on the floor, try to bring your knee to the wall. Switch and assess the other side.

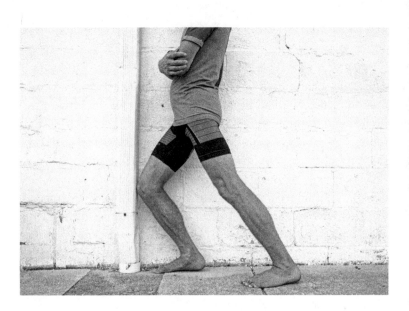

Hip extension assessment

Lie flat on a table and hug your knee (as your other leg hangs over the end of the table). When you hug your knee, does the other thigh elevate off the table? Assess both sides.

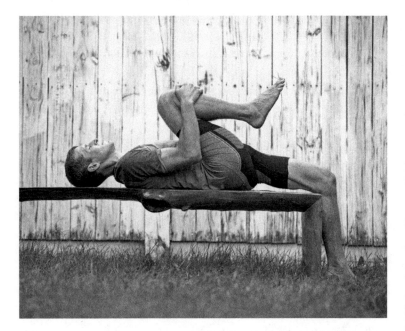

Quad length test (affecting hip mobility)
While lying prone (on your belly), bend the knee of one leg and bring your heel to your butt. Assess both sides.

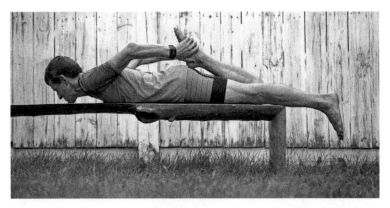

Prone

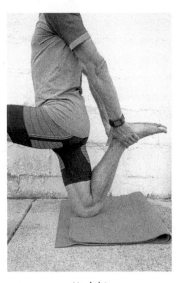

Upright

Range-of-motion drills

Six-position foot walk

This simple exercise snack works the small muscles of your feet and ankles, and assists with balance and foot strength. Barefoot, preferably, walk in the following manner whenever you can (for instance, when walking the dog), initially for short distances. Walk:

1. On the outsides of your feet (inversion).
2. On the insides of your feet (eversion).
3. Toes pointing outward (Charlie Chaplin style).
4. Toes pointing inward (pigeon-toed).
5. On the balls of your feet, backward.
6. On your heels (you may need shoes, if not barefoot adapted).

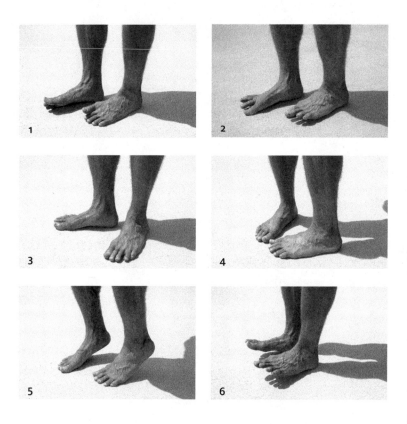

The squat—rediscovering one of the most basic positions

Kids squat naturally and easily. Adults typically say, "I'm not built like a child anymore, and can't get into that position." It's true that your body geometry is different, but to reclaim your flexibility and mobility, you still need to be able to squat.

The prime movers in squatting are the muscles around the hips and knees, but all joints below the belly button (hip, knee, ankle,

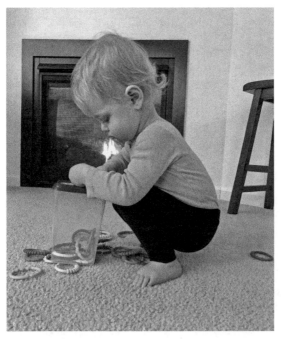

Looks perfect! Just do your best to rediscover this.

foot) and most of the spine need stability and mobility for a proper squat.

Align your feet comfortably under your hips (or slightly wider). Then move directly to a full squat. As you do so, try to maintain a good, flexible posture, with your:

- Head and thoracic spine upright.
- Lumbar spine neutral, not hyperextended.
- Arms in front and shoulder blades "tucked." (Think of putting your shoulder blades into your back pockets.)
- Hips mobile, sitting back as if tapping a chair behind you with your glutes (but not sitting).
- Knees tracking directly over the toes. Use a resistance band around the knees, and apply outward pressure.
- Shins close to perpendicular to the ground. (Your knees shouldn't extend over your toes.)
- Weight on your heels, and heels remaining on the ground.

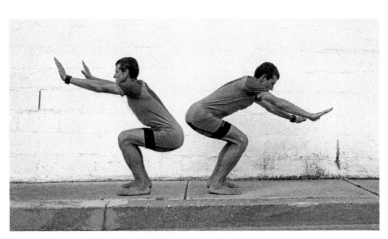

Which does your squat look like? Aim for the picture on the left.

Progress to a deep squat ("ass to grass," as they say). If your heels come off the ground, place a book or two under the heels and work on gradually removing them. This will help the mobility of the ankle. Vary the foot position. The goal is to hang out comfortably in a deep squat for a few minutes. But if you have any discomfort, restriction, or tightness in the knees, stop when your thighs are perpendicular to the ground. It may take time to work into a full squat.

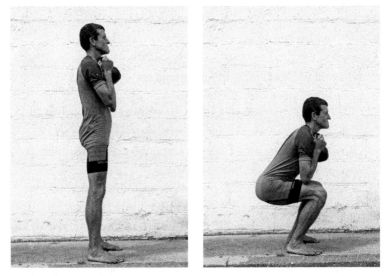

Or load yourself with a kettlebell, in an exercise called the goblet squat.

The wall squat

To further assess the mobility of the thoracic spine, stand with your toes close to the wall (or, ideally, right up to it). Raise your arms high overhead, and try to drop down into your basic squat. Can you get your thighs to a level parallel with the ground? Can you drop your bottom all the way down? Do this routine especially if your upper back is restricting you.

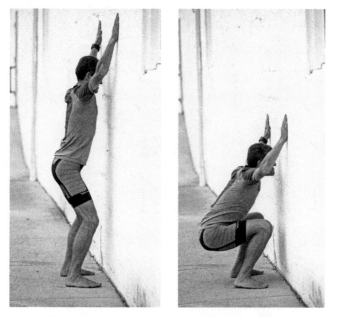

By working on upper body, hip, and ankle mobility,
you'll be able to do a wall squat.

Floor sitting

We should all be exploring the ground whenever we can. We can do this (without spending extra time in our day) by sitting on the floor. Here are five floor-sitting positions, in addition to the deep squat, that will greatly boost your flexibility and range of motion:

Kneeling. Lost from most Western cultures, this requires quad and ankle mobility. Use a pad for your butt and knees if you're uncomfortable. As an interim measure, try kneeling on one leg while doing some of your work. This will build hip and core stability.

Long sitting. Sit with both legs extended, straight out. This builds hamstring mobility. Tuck one leg in for variation. *Cross-legged*, or "Indian style." Tight IT bands and piriformis will cause the knees to elevate. Work to keep the knees lower. As a variation, place the soles of your feet together.

Side sitting. Place one leg in internal rotation and the other in external rotation. Change sides, and assess tightness and symmetry. This can be challenging.

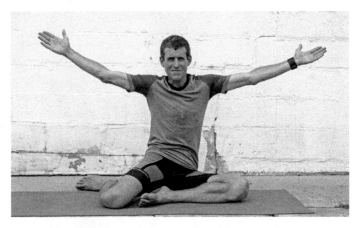

Upper body mobility

T-spine foam roll

Move into these positions slowly, with diaphragm breathing, to open up your thoracic spine.

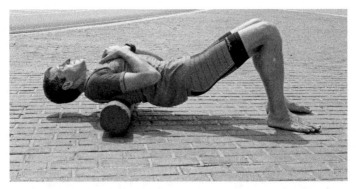

Move slowly up and down each segment, while deep breathing.

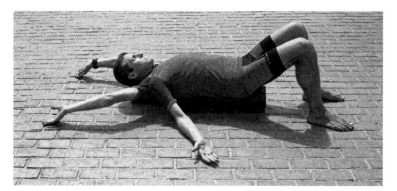
Move shoulders and arms as if making a snow angel

Supple hips

The windshield wiper progression

This exercise generates good internal and external rotation of the hips, with glute firing and hip extension. It's especially good for golfers, who need at least 25 degrees of internal rotation of the lead hip on the backswing, and the same on the other hip on follow-through. (The average PGA golfer has 45 degrees of internal rotation.) If you don't have this range, you'll end up compensating elsewhere in the kinetic chain.

- Lie on the floor, with back flat, arms stretched straight out, knees bent at 90 degrees, and heels on the floor.
- In a slow, smooth motion, sweep your knees back and forth, to the right and then to the left, in a windshield wiper motion. Keep your shoulder blades on the floor, with arms extended. Repeat ten to fifteen times.

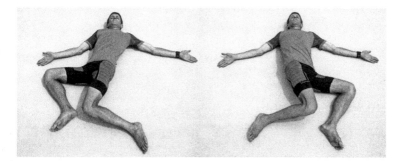

Heel raises

Foot control is essential to running, and helpful in all activities. Simply balance on one foot, raise up on the ball, and finish by loading weight onto the big toe and rotating the lower leg slightly toward the big toe (to get maximum plantar flexion). This is the full range of motion employed when walking and running correctly. Slowly lower yourself, with control, to the start position. If you can, knock off fifty to one hundred of these on each foot daily. Progress from the ground to lowering from a step.

Single-leg sit-to-stand

This simple and revealing exercise can be done while sitting in your office chair:

- Sit on the chair with your feet flat on the ground.
- Select one leg, and elevate slowly on that leg, with arms extended overhead. Pause on the ball of the foot, then lower yourself slowly, in a controlled manner. Don't let your knee collapse inward.

Single-leg hop

Another simple (but somewhat challenging) stability drill is to simply hop on one foot ten times. If you're unable to do this without pain, or are wobbly, return to the single-leg sit drill above, and progress to this.

Fire hydrants

This move assists hip mobility and strength in both extension and abduction, which are essential for running. On all fours, elevate

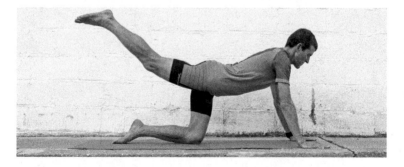

and extend one leg, and draw large circles with it, clockwise, then counterclockwise. For an additional challenge, extend the opposite arm directly forward into the "bird dog" pose.

There are three tests of hip, glute, and core stability. Hold each of these positions for one minute:

Bridge single leg
Lying on your back, tuck one knee to the chest and tighten the glutes. Then "bridge" (elevate) your core upward.

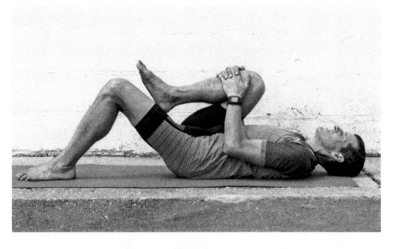

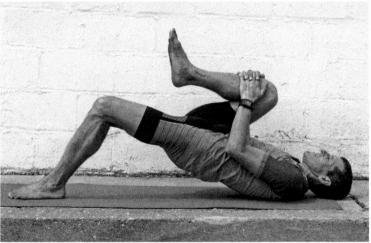

Plank

Lie prone on a mat or the floor. Place your forearms on the mat, elbows under shoulders. Place the legs together. Elevate your body into a straight line. Hold for thirty to sixty seconds.

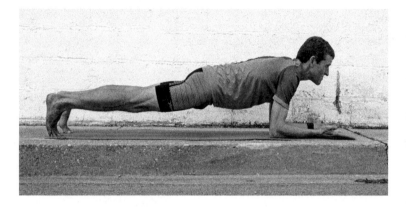

Side plank

Lie on your side on a mat or the floor. Place your forearm on the mat, perpendicular to the body. Place the upper leg on top of the lower leg and straighten your knees and hips. Raise your body up until it is rigid. Hold for thirty to sixty seconds. Repeat on the opposite side.

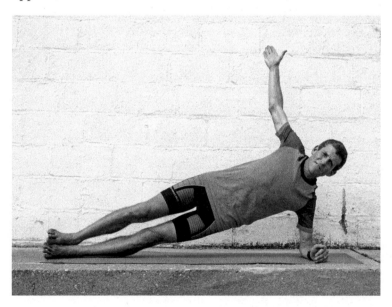

Video assistance

My colleague Jay Dicharry and I demonstrate some excellent assessments and corrections for improving range of motion and stability in "Are You Ready to Go Minimal? 3 Self-assessment tests with Jay Dicharry," on the videos page of runforyourlifebook.com.

Once you have progressed by mixing these movements into your day, the final exercise is the Turkish Getup, which incorporates nearly all of the preceding exercises. This sequence (see the video by this name) will help you visually piece together this timeless exercise.

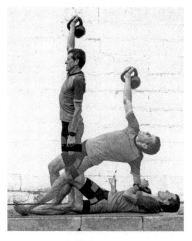 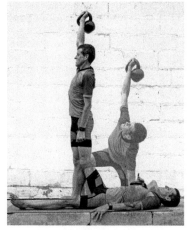

Turkish Getup
up move

Reverse to slowly
go down

CHAPTER 9

Eating to Go the Distance: Nutrition and Health

People are fed by the food industry, which pays no attention to health, and are treated by the health industry, which pays no attention to food.

—WENDELL BERRY,
author and sixth-generation Kentucky farmer

MYTH: *Eating fat makes you fat.*

FACT: *Sugars, processed carbohydrates, and a "low-fat" diet can lead to bonking, inflammation, and weight gain. Healthy fat, by contrast, provides long-term stamina and health, curtails hunger, and aids in weight loss.*

By now, your running form has improved, you have better footwear, and you're on the path to building your endurance engine. In order to maintain and optimize that engine and boost performance, it's time to check on the quality (and quantity) of your fuel. You might even want to consider a fuel upgrade.

We'll explore the specific implications for our diet in the next chapter, but first let's take a look at what happens when food enters our bodies and begins its long and complicated transformation into fuel, body fat, waste products, and sometimes even forward movement.

The units of energy that power us are commonly measured in calories. The conventional wisdom of "energy balance" says that if *calories in* equal *calories out,* then your body weight remains stable.

But this deduction is flawed. Clearly, it takes more energy to maintain vigorous work than to rest or to sleep. But not all calories going in are identical, nor are all of those consumed calories digested, stored, or drawn upon for combustion in the same way. And food has an annoying tendency to morph and migrate to unexpected places, and park itself where we don't want it.

OVEREATING AND UNDERNOURISHED

Part of the problem is that our food isn't delivering the nutrition that we really need.

In medical school, I believed (as many doctors still do) that a high-carbohydrate, low-fat diet was essential for athletic performance and health, and that exercise was the key to weight control. That's what we were taught, and what the world believed. Like other young, near-tireless athletes, I began each day with a huge bowl of cereal and skim milk for breakfast, an energy bar or bread for a morning snack, and more carbs for lunch. After meetings, I hoarded any energy bars or muffins left behind on the conference table. Then I gobbled up a pound of spaghetti for dinner, devoured more cereal before bed, and awoke at two in the morning for an expedition to the kitchen to eat more cereal.

My running colleagues and I got away with consuming high-carb diets because we exercised athletically, and believed that if the fire is hot enough it can burn (metabolize) anything. My race times were reasonably good, partly because I understood pacing and training. And my weight remained stable, so I assumed my diet was on the right track. I urged others to follow my example. As a doctor and a competitive runner, I even promoted pre-race "carbo loading" dinners.

Except for a distracting problem. I couldn't seem to shake a perpetual state of hunger, and an unexplainable sense of fatigue. I didn't realize it at the time, but I was on the path to type 2 diabetes. My blood labs showed that I already had the condition known as prediabetcs.

CALORIE BALANCE DOES NOT COMPUTE

I had carefully measured and recorded my activity levels, but I began to wonder: was it possible that my fatigue and hunger had more to do with *diet* than with how active I was? Nutrition was one ingredient in my performance cocktail that I figured I could adjust. But I knew of no alternative to the diet regimen I was on.

That's when I became intrigued, then obsessed, with what happens to us when we consume food. I tumbled down the scientific rabbit hole of physiology and metabolism, and devoured age-old and emerging studies on nutrition, energy balance, obesity, the hormones that affect appetite, fat storage, and the urge to exercise. I sought out experts, queried and observed members of the military, chatted with patients who came through our hospital, and engaged the citizens in our community.

WHERE DOES YOUR SUGAR GO?

So, what was going on? How *does* the food we eat affect how we feel and what happens in our bodies?

Our bodies demand that glucose levels in the blood remain within a narrow range. That level is regulated by a complex interplay of hormones, chemicals, signaling proteins, and glucose disposal pathways, which in turn are signaled by environmental factors such as our level of exertion, the types of food we eat, stress, sleep, and even the microbes in our gut. For most of us, moments after we consume refined carbohydrates or a sugared drink, the sugar level in our blood rises. The muscles, brain, and other organs use this glucose as their fuel, and if there's an immediate demand for energy from these organs, they can directly utilize some of the recently ingested glucose.

But the blood can't store more than a *teaspoon* of glucose, so there's not a lot of buffer for maintaining blood sugar levels within a narrow healthy range. When the blood glucose level rises after eating a breakfast bar, for instance, the pancreas releases the hormone insulin, which drives that sugar from the bloodstream and into our muscles and liver, in the form of glycogen.

These "glycogen tanks" within the liver and muscles aren't very large, either. If you ate your breakfast bar before doing much activity, those tanks are likely already full.

When the glycogen tanks are full, the liver converts additional incoming sugars to a type of fat called triglycerides, through a process called *de novo lipogenesis*. Much of those triglycerides are then stored in the cells of our adipose tissue, or (long-term) visceral fat, also known as belly fat.

If you are *insulin sensitive,* your body responds quickly and appropriately to the rise in blood sugar and insulin, and vigorously manages the sugar/energy balance. But if the incoming sugar just keeps on coming, the triglyceride fat builds up faster than the liver can ship it out, and the liver can no longer respond normally to insulin's signals.

This is the beginning of *insulin resistance.* Now, in response to persistent sugar elevation, the pancreas has no choice but to *further* elevate insulin levels in a desperate attempt to overcome the resistance. A vicious carb- and insulin-driven cycle begins. That's why the body and mind of the insulin-resistant person are persistently hijacked by fatigue and hunger. A simplified version of a complex progression summarizes this endless loop:

More sugar → more insulin → more insulin resistance →
more calorie/fat storage → less energy available to muscles →
more hunger → more sugar . . .

Fructose (found in high concentration in processed foods and drinks) compounds the problem, because it can be metabolized only in the liver; the quantities and concentrations of fructose that we typically consume quickly inundate the liver. Essentially, fructose metabolism is not as well regulated as glucose metabolism—it appears to have less "metabolic flexibility"—and tends to force the body into building fat.

If you are insulin resistant (carbohydrate intolerant, or prediabetic), the active muscles are deprived of the energy they seek. That's when the appetite—sensing insufficient energy available for use by the muscles—becomes supercharged with an urgent drive to *eat,* as it attempts to compensate for the *perceived* lack of fuel.

After a decade or more of this "normal" abuse, the pancreas may lose its ability to compensate, and the body can no longer control blood sugar levels. Those with escalating insulin resistance risk developing a fatty liver, which we'll discuss below.

DIABETES: A REVERSIBLE PANDEMIC

The incidence in America of type 2 diabetes is near-epidemic. But few are aware of the condition known as prediabetes—the state of insulin resistance and higher-than-normal blood glucose levels that aren't yet high enough to be labeled as type 2 diabetes. With unchecked prediabetes, insulin levels continue to rise, while increasing amounts of sugar are converted to visceral fat. Our typically late diagnosis of prediabetes is akin to waiting until a large, visible tumor appears before thinking about cancer.

Most folks with prediabetes don't realize they have it, and are unaware of its long-term risks: fully developed diabetes, heart attack, stroke, and even Alzheimer's. A recent article in the *Journal of the American Medical Association* reports that more than half of adult Americans—and increasing numbers elsewhere—have diabetes or prediabetes. And the Centers for Disease Control and Prevention (CDC) project that if current trends continue unaddressed, nearly half of people with prediabetes will develop type 2 diabetes within five years. We are now seeing this condition in children and no longer label it "adult diabetes."

TOO MUCH TREATMENT, NOT ENOUGH CARE

Every day I witness at least one case of prediabetes that has been dismissed as "normal" or has been missed altogether, despite the ease with which it can be detected. Any change in body configuration in the direction of accumulating abdominal fat is a preliminary sign. To put it bluntly: if you're a male, you should be able to see your private parts while standing in the shower. For women, the circumference of your waist shouldn't be greater than that of your chest. Or simply multiply your waist circumference by two. It should be less than your height.

Sadly, I see too many insulin-resistant, prediabetic patients

THE INSULIN RESISTANCE CONTINUUM

| Carbohydrate Intolerant | | Carbohydrate Tolerant |

INSULIN RESISTANT
Type-2 diabetes
Metabolic syndrome
Obesity
Expanding waistline

INSULIN SENSITIVITY
Athletes
Normal BMI

We all fit somewhere along this spectrum.
Most of us move to the left as we age.

who advance to full-blown diabetes without a health care provider having ever urged them to modify their diet or lifestyle beyond suggesting that they "eat less and exercise more." Even when care providers do intervene, they often send patients in the wrong direction, typically by recommending a low-fat, high-carb diet—the opposite of what most need. Indeed, the American Diabetes Association's "Create Your Plate" dietary guidelines don't restrict carbs and reduce the saturated fats. And the current CDC/AMA/ADA-supported site *So . . . Do I Have Prediabetes?* doesn't even suggest reducing carb intake, despite these groups' recognition in their own papers that carbohydrates are the main drivers of high blood glucose levels. Again and again, dietary fat remains the perceived culprit. So what are we to replace the fat with? Carbohydrates? No wonder remission from diabetes is rarely seen.

SUGAR AND CARBS

Medical literature has established that the prevalence of diabetes and the development of prediabetes correlate with the duration and degree of exposure to sugar and refined carbohydrates. But the food, pharmaceutical, and medical industries are slow to catch up. They have little interest in reversing diabetes, because ongoing treatment for it as a chronic disease forms a lucrative revenue stream. Better to offer a lifetime of treatment than a cure.

Diabetes isn't the only condition to fear from sugar. Long before diabetes develops, high insulin and blood sugar levels can trigger inflammation, which contributes to vessel stiffening and development of plaque and "intimal thickening" in the inner lining of the arteries. (The oxidation of manufactured oils, including vegetable oils, amplifies this process.)

This thickening and stiffening can inhibit optimal blood flow to the heart and brain, and (even more dangerously) the plaque can rupture and cause heart arrhythmia or stroke. The body's attempt to "heal" the rupturing plaque can cause a thrombus, or clot, which can also block an artery. Contrary to decades of conventional wisdom (and increasingly confirmed population studies, and meta-analyses of pooled trials and prospective trials), atherosclerosis doesn't result from consumption of dietary fat. The most likely suspect is inflammation driven by insulin resistance. The recent PURE (Prospective Urban Rural Epidemiology) study in eighteen countries with 130,000 patients again confirmed this.

THERE'S EVEN MORE TO (NOT) LOOK FORWARD TO . . .

High blood sugar levels and manufactured fats (i.e., vegetable oils) also produce nasty metabolic by-products that drive inflammation and further contribute to cardiovascular disease. These include *reactive oxidative species* (ROS), and also *advanced glycated endproducts* (AGES), or glycations, in which glucose binds with proteins on the outer surface membranes of cells. Once the glucose is stuck onto the cell membrane, it can't get off. This makes the cells less pliable and more vulnerable to damage and premature aging.

This process (and the inflammatory cascade from persistently high insulin levels) eventually leads to what is called *metabolic syndrome,* the precursor to diabetes and its grim manifestations: blindness, atherosclerosis, high blood pressure, heart attacks, strokes,

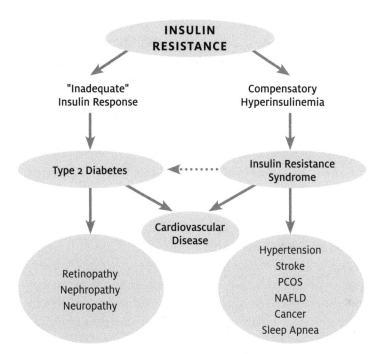

In 1980, Gerald Reaven identified "Syndrome X," which is nowadays called metabolic syndrome. The path on the right summarizes the clinical syndromes related to the inflammatory and hormonal dysfunction of persistent high insulin levels. The path on the left follows the development of hyperglycemia. Driving it all is insulin resistance.

kidney damage, impotence, loss of feeling in the feet, and dementia. Metabolic syndrome might better be termed something more descriptive but suitably alarming, such as "insulin resistance/carbohydrate intolerance" or, more accurately, "hyperinsulinemia."

DESTINATION: LIVER

A hundred years ago, Americans ate 4 pounds of added sugar a year. Now each of us consumes over 125 pounds of sugar, much of it as fructose in sugar-sweetened beverages. Add to that our annual per capita consumption of 140 pounds of processed flour, which is quickly converted to glucose during digestion. This is the direct cause of a condition known as fatty liver, or nonalcoholic fatty liver disease (NAFLD)—which in turn drives diabetes.

The physiology of the insulin resistance and fatty liver disease relationship is not fully understood, but the results are clinically significant. Now unfortunate victims of this sugar-driven disease are lining up for liver transplants, without being offered measures to reverse it, nor knowledge of how they acquired it. (It may be instructive that food producers create foie gras, the delicacy made from the fatty liver of geese, by force-feeding the birds starch, an easily digestible form of carbohydrate.)

WHICH SUGAR IS WHICH?

Table sugar and sodas are a mix of glucose and fructose. Fruit is primarily fructose, but tends to be absorbed more slowly because it travels with fiber. Flour is mostly glucose—thus the high "glycemic index" of flour products. High fructose corn syrup (HFCS, a staple ingredient in soft drinks) is a mixture of both, and present in *many* foods, not just soft drinks.

Almost every cell in our body can utilize glucose. Fructose, however, because of its structure, needs to pass through the liver. This means that fructose has a lower glycemic index, because the absorption happens more slowly. But this isn't a good thing: a high fructose load on the liver overwhelms the metabolic processes, causing fat to accumulate in the liver. This may be the first stage of insulin resistance.

BACK TO THE LIVER

Most people, including many physicians, dismiss "fatty liver" as a largely innocuous condition stemming from *being* fat, or from *consuming* too much dietary fat. (More accurately, one might describe NAFLD as "carby liver" because it originates from insulin resistance and the conversion of excess sugar and carbohydrates that are converted to triglycerides.) But the condition is much more insidious, and its effects can be quite rapid. Dr. Robert Lustig recently published a study comparing the effect of fructose intake in children. Compared to children who consumed the same number of calories of better-quality carbohydrates, the high fructose consumption group showed markers of liver dysfunction and metabolic syndrome in just ten days.

The only effective treatment for fatty liver is to short-circuit its causes—meaning at the source, by reducing the ingestion of carbs, especially fructose, and lowering body weight by 10 percent. Fortunately, fatty liver can be readily diagnosed: it appears in a panel of liver enzymes as a rise in the transaminases GGT, AST, and ALT. It is often picked up "incidentally" during an ultrasound or CT scan of the liver.

So what are the early indicators of insulin resistance that a doctor might look for in a clinical setting? We have known for some time that one's *waist* is more important than one's *weight*. It's healthy, in fact, to carry a certain amount of fat under your skin. This is metabolically active "brown fat." Belly fat, or "white fat," is a different beast, as it indicates that you are storing fat in and around the internal organs, such as the liver and heart. In the presence of obesity, a high TG/HDL ratio, a high fasting or post-meal insulin or glucose level, or any hemoglobin A1c reading (a key diabetes screen) higher than 5.5 (the ideal is below 5.0) is also cause for concern. Fatigue, constant hunger, an irritable GI tract, feelings of low blood sugar or "crashes"—or any chronic pain or inflammatory disorder—are additional flags for insulin resistance/carbohydrate intolerance (metabolic syndrome). But insulin resistance can be detected even *before* waist circumference expands, in the form of fat accumulation under the mandible, particularly in normal-weight people.

A CHERISHED ADDICTION

One of the biggest challenges in treating diabetes and obesity-related diseases is that sugars hit the happy center of the brain. Dr. Lustig has illuminated how fructose in particular stimulates the nucleus accumbens, or "hedonic pathway," by creating a tasty reward, habituation, and possible dependence that parallels that of alcohol or other drug addiction. We eat carbs for comfort, as a handy after-school snack, a nightly treat, or simply to relieve stress.

Like the hourly hit of a cigarette, we get rewarded and become habituated. Nutritionists even encourage "small, frequent meals," which are almost always low-fat and high-carb. Fruit juice is a culprit, too. But implicating the citrus industry in this public health disaster would be political suicide. Remember your grandmother's juice glasses? They were the size of a shot glass.

The public health implications of this are immense. If you consider the role that the sugar and flour industries play in our society and economy, curtailing the consumption of these products presents a sizable political challenge. As with any substance of abuse, combating the obesity epidemic will require proactive social and legislative measures to reduce sugar consumption. As with dieting in general, as we will discuss, *willpower alone cannot be relied upon as a sustainable regulator of behavior.*

OBESITY: EGG FIRST, OR CHICKEN?

Obesity is a disorder of abnormal fat accumulation, in most cases driven by eating more carbohydrates than an insulin-resistant body can handle. The excess insulin generated from overeating of carbs begins to act as an accelerator, in essence, for the growth of body fat. We may continue to argue over whether obesity (defined as a body mass index greater than 30) is a disease as such, but it is an important *marker* for all the other metabolic diseases we see today.

Is BMI the sole indicator of insulin resistance? Dr. Lustig estimates that 40 percent of U.S. adults with a normal BMI have some spectrum of this condition, and are referred to as TOFI ("Thin on the Outside, Fat on the Inside"). And some who are overweight do not have insulin resistance. It is possible to be obese and healthy, with normal metabolic functioning, but this is less common. Most college football players would be considered obese, judging by BMI alone, but they are often metabolically healthy. At the same time, 40 percent of *non-obese* Americans have early or full-blown metabolic syndrome.

Obesity is commonly dismissed as a product of being gluttonous and lazy. But it's not the behavior of overeating and sitting on one's butt that drives obesity. *It's the obesity that drives the behavior.*

How does this work? The condition of insulin resistance begets the drive to eat. As incoming carb calories are converted to fat, the desire to move or exercise is reduced, which begets more insulin resistance, which increases hunger—all in a negative feedback loop.

One powerful actor here is the dysfunction of the hunger gauge—the brain's appestat, which tells us when we are hungry and full. Leptin, a recently discovered satiety hormone, is released by our fat cells and signals the feeling of fullness. We now know that leptin brain signaling is inhibited by insulin. So for our appestat to reset at a healthy level, we need the high insulin levels to go away. A hormone called ghrelin (think of your stomach growling) is another satiety hormone secreted mostly by the stomach, and it also regulates the appestat.

Thus obesity results largely from hormonal dysregulation and insulin resistance, through complex processes. It's not a dysfunction of energy balance. It may be instructive that insulin resistance also "travels with" the hormonal shifts of pregnancy, menopause, and sleeplessness, in similar ways.

THE WORLD IS GROWING IN SIZE . . .

For most modern humans, as discussed prior, a portion of the sugars and fats we consume is turned into belly fat. Even if the rate of conversion is modest, the effects accumulate over time. The incidence of obesity in the United States has tripled since 1970, and our current generation is projected to be the first to live shorter functional lives than their parents did. And as developing countries around the world catch up economically and culturally with America, their rates of obesity are catching up, too. Fast-food restaurants are everywhere—Cinnabon, McDonald's, KFC, Cheesecake Factory, and others—all with colorful advertising and modern, fast-food prices and appeal.

Ironically, we see this occurring even in the Middle East, for example, where traditional cuisine is among the healthiest in the world. For centuries, meals there have been prepared from simple and inexpensive ingredients, including marvelous mixes of legumes, spices, meat, and small amounts of whole grains. It's being replaced by fast food. And as temperatures in the region trend toward the brutally hot, most people take refuge in the comfort of air-conditioning—increasing sedentary behavior and compounding the risk of obesity, diabetes, and heart disease. Similarly, the obesity and prediabetes epidemics are spreading to China, India, and other countries, where healthful traditional diets are being swapped out for junk food that comes at generally lower cost and offers lower nutritive value.

SALT'S NOT AT FAULT

Sugar presents an even greater risk than the other white crystal that we are routinely cautioned against consuming too much of—salt. Sodium is prevalent in our diets, thanks to industrially processed foods, yet these same food products frequently contain added sugars and processed oils as well, which studies have associated even *more* closely with hypertension and cardiometabolic risk. Salt has been exonerated of the peril once attributed to it, meaning that it's time we shifted our attention to the real culprit—sugar, the white crystal now of greatest concern. In yet another medical research flip-flop, a diet too low in sodium is now associated with *higher* risk of cardiometabolic disease.

SIX YEARS A (CEREAL) FREE MAN

I haven't had a bowl of cereal in six years. I now eat two or three meals daily, always including a good quantity of healthy fat and adequate protein. I am seldom hungry, and enjoy sustained energy throughout the day. My body weight is constant and my key lipid (cholesterol subtype) levels and inflammatory markers (such as hsCRP, an indicator of blood vessel damage) are optimal—far better than they were when I was on the high-carb diet. My HDL (good cholesterol) has doubled, and is now over 100 mg/dl. My coronary artery calcium score—arguably the best marker for any vascular disease—is zero. I even subjected myself to a test that measures telomere length. This novel marker of how our cells' DNA ages pegs me as a thirty-five-year-old, though I'm fifty-one.

I don't fear that I might bonk during marathons, and I *feel* healthier overall. That being said, my twenty years of eating a high-carb diet and the resulting high insulin production (and progressive insulin resistance) has left me now with little more than a trickle of pancreatic function. I have prediabetes and extremely low insulin levels. But by avoiding carbs and living healthfully, I've lowered my HGB A1c (a marker of average blood sugar) from 6.3 to 5.5. A small serving of simple carbs sends my sugar to near 200 mg/dl, so I need to restrict carbs for the rest of my life. I'm doing this now, and still running marathons with vigor.

As one individual, I'm a pretty small sample size. But I've assisted many runners and nonrunners who have insulin resistance in shifting their diets to low carb, and have seen their key risk markers and health indicators improve, along with their feeling of well-being.

I had a patient whose blood sugar was out of control—persistently over 500 mg/dl—and she had increased her insulin injections to more than 500 units a day. A healthy body requires about 20 to 25 units. But the added insulin was not driving her blood sugar level down. She felt horrible. Incredibly, she was trapped in the regimen of conventional medical treatment that persists today: give such patients even *more* insulin, to try to overcome the extreme resistance.

My patient hadn't heard of the alternative: get rid of the sugar (the fire) in her diet, which was driving the elevated sugar in her blood (the smoke). She cut out sugar and began eating healthful and satiating meals, and within three days she had reduced her insulin injections to 40 units (long-acting), once daily. After a week, her sugar levels were near normal, and she is buoyed by the belief that she can be well again. A bit of discipline and hope can go a long way in the long term.

THE BIG FAT LIE

So, what about cholesterol? Books and conferences have been devoted to debating its value and its peril. The perception that high levels of total cholesterol were associated with cardiovascular disease originated in the 1950s, when a high-profile researcher named Ancel Keys drew a flawed correlation between dietary fat and the risk of heart disease, based on partial data from six selected countries. The resulting "diet-heart hypothesis" posited logically, but incorrectly, that *dietary* fat and cholesterol elevated the levels of *blood* fat and cholesterol, and therefore led directly to clogging of the arteries.

This hypothesis, in turn, informed the creation of the ill-conceived 1977 *Dietary Goals for the United States,* which birthed the first version of the *Dietary Guidelines for Americans.* These were illustrated by the ubiquitous "Food Pyramid," which succeeded at convincing Americans to consume less fat and more carbohydrate. This was replaced in 2011 by "My Plate," a simpler graphic that encouraged a similar mistaken balance of foods. (See more on this in the next chapter.)

CHANGE IN DIETARY COMPOSITION IN RELATION TO OBESITY PREVALENCE (1971–2010)

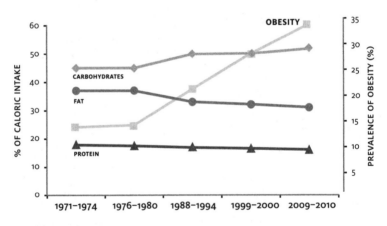

ADAPTED FROM: FLEGAL, K.M. *INT J OBES* 1998; HEDLE, A.A. ET AL., *JAMA* 2004 291(23): 2847–50; FLEGAL K.M. ET AL., *JAMA.* 2012 307(5): 491–7

Dietary and blood cholesterol, it turns out, are not the bad guys at the crime scene of inflamed arteries. They are merely suspicious-looking bystanders.

Saturated fats in the blood come from two sources: the saturated fat that you eat (odd-chain fats), and the saturated fat produced in the liver (even-chain fats). Metabolically, these two categories of fats behave quite differently. The liver-generated fats are the most dangerous, because they end up as belly fat (visceral fat, or white fat). What Ancel Keys and generations of health professionals were unaware of, or disregarded, was that *this liver-generated fat doesn't originate from fat that we ingest.* It is produced by the liver when we take in *carbohydrates, fructose,* and *alcohol.* It is this fat—not the ingested, dietary kind—that increases risk for diabetes and heart attacks.

I believe that our adherence, whether inadvertent or intentional, to the government's guidelines is to blame for the fact that we have an obese nation—one that has grown fatter and sicker with each generation since 1980.

RETHINKING THE OTHER "C" WORD

Cholesterol, a lipid molecule, is present in every cell membrane of the body, and is essential for almost every endocrine function we have. It is insoluble in water, so it must be transported in a lipoprotein. This is where the terms *HDL* (high-density lipoprotein) and *LDL* (low-density lipoprotein) come in.

In popular usage, HDL has been described as "good" cholesterol (because, theoretically, it scavenges up plaque) and LDL as "bad" cholesterol (because it's thought to clog arteries). But this distinction is misleading. Indeed, many of those who have suffered a first heart attack have LDL levels in the "safe" range, and many of those with LDL levels in the "unsafe" range will never have a heart attack. When looked at in isolation (outside rare genetic predispositions), a high LDL cholesterol level alone carries little risk.

For a moment, set aside LDL. The dance between carbohydrates and the liver affects other elements of cholesterol levels, too. In a standard lipid panel there's one blood test ratio in particular that can reasonably tell if you are at risk for prediabetes, diabetes, or a heart attack. The *triglyceride ratio* (TG/HDL) is calculated by dividing your triglyceride level (TG) by your HDL level. This should be close to or less than 1. A ratio creeping toward 4 or 5 portends bad news. The total cholesterol to HDL ratio is also useful with a target of less than 3. I see far too many panels with ratios that are 4 and above.

What causes a poor TG/HDL ratio? When blood sugar (and corresponding triglyceride) levels rise, the body tries to "clean up" the abundance of triglycerides by using HDL cholesterol (the "good" kind) to carry the triglycerides back to the liver, where they came from. Thus a low HDL level combined with a high TG reading indicates liver overdrive, and is a clear early sign of carbohydrate intolerance and insulin resistance.

The LDL story is complex and not fully understood. The lipoprotein is the vehicle for the cholesterol (the passengers). It's really this lipoprotein vehicle that we care about, as the passengers are merely along for the ride.

There are many varieties of lipoproteins, across a spectrum. The LDL-C that your doctor orders and interprets is a calculated number (thus "C") from at least five unique LDLs; it provides an aggregated estimate of the LDL cholesterol, without regard to the number and size of particles.

The LDL particle size is what makes the difference: a small number of large particles is good. But an abundance of small-sized particles correlates with insulin resistance, low HDL, and high triglycerides. Small-sized LDL particles are prone to oxidation and can easily penetrate the endothelial lining of our blood vessels, amplifying inflammation. When it comes to LDL and risk, you want the big vehicles, or particles. (Two thousand passengers riding in twenty one-hundred-passenger buses is safer than two thousand passengers riding in a thousand sports cars.)

Therapy with statin drugs can lower the LDL-C to an industry-established target, yet this still may not reduce cardiovascular disease risk. A patient may have a high number of small-sized particles yet a low LDL-C reading. This "discordance," as it is known, is remarkably common among diabetics and the insulin resistant.

Simply put, it's better to take care of your health than to take drugs. Pay attention to the circumference of your waist, and your sugar tolerance. Your TG/HDL ratio is a strong indicator of where you are in terms of insulin resistance.

GOOD NEWS AWAITS

The good news is that prediabetes (and even type 2 diabetes) can often be reversed through changes in diet. Improvement will be further leveraged by increased physical activity. When a tasty toxin such as sugar becomes acceptable, accessible, and affordable, public health suffers.

It was thirty years after medical studies decisively illuminated the dangers of tobacco that action was taken. Now taxes, restrictions on public use, minimum age of purchase, public awareness, and illness and death have effectively reduced the number of smokers. We must treat our toxic food environment the same way. In the history of public health, no problem affecting more than half of the population has been successfully dealt with by "treatment." The only solution is prevention. For this, your diet, which is discussed in the next chapter, matters most.

DRILLS

Carbohydrate intolerance test

My brilliant colleague Dr. Phil Maffetone has developed a simple and effective way to determine if you are carbohydrate intolerant—which many of us are. The "2 week test" is not a diet, really, nor is it onerously restrictive, but it can indicate if you are suffering what may be the most overlooked epidemic of our time. You can learn more about it at runforyourlifebook.com.

Baseline lab work—to place you ahead of the curve

I urge even those who consider themselves healthy to have basic lab tests done, in order to establish a baseline for future comparison. All of the tests below are common and affordable, and are generally covered by insurance under an annual physical checkup.

Basic Tests
- Complete metabolic panel, which includes liver function and enzymes, kidney function, and sugar levels
- Standard lipid panel, with attention to the TG/HDL ratio and TC/HDL ratio
- Hemoglobin A1c
- Vitamin D and B_{12}
- Thyroid panel
- Blood count (CBC)
- Ferritin (iron stores)
- hsCRP
- Uric acid

Second-Level Tests for Higher Risk Groups
- Fasted glucose and insulin tests (before breakfast, for instance)
- 75–100 gram Glucose Tolerance Test (GTT): glucose and insulin tests one to two hours after glucose drink
- Advanced lipid profile (available from LabCorps). This test provides the important LDL particle size and number. (You want large size and small number.)

- Coronary artery calcium (CAC) score, to quantify your coronary artery disease (about $100 at imaging centers)

Securing the test results is one thing. Finding a knowledgeable health care provider is even more important—someone who can help you interpret the results, especially taking into account your unique circumstances.

Create a sugar-free home or workplace

Just this year at my hospital, Jefferson Medical Center, we became the first hospital in the state to eliminate sugar-sweetened beverages for patients, staff, and visitors. My children are teenagers and not on a low-carb diet, but we do not have sugar-sweetened beverages, including juice, in our home.

CHAPTER 10

What's for Dinner:
Setting Your Meal Course

Status quo, you know, is Latin for "the mess we're in."
—RONALD REAGAN

Your health and likely your life span will be determined by the proportion of fat versus sugar you burn over a lifetime.
—DR. RON ROSEDALE

MYTH: *There are healthy and unhealthy diets.*

FACT: *Diets are not* healthy. *People are either* healthy *or* unhealthy.

MYTH: *Medical experts and government officials, over time, have figured out what's best for us in terms of our nutrition.*

FACT: *Disturbingly, the government's dietary recommendations may be contributing to the growth of prediabetes, type 2 diabetes, obesity, and chronic diseases.*

Ah yes . . . diets.

Don't do it. Don't diet. Nearly every "diet" with a name is little more than a fad, or it has debatable efficacy.

Why do people following Weight Watchers fail to lose weight

for the long term? Look up their "Points" list. If overweight folks consistently eat bananas and mangos (which have been granted their desirable zero Points ranking), most will gain weight. I was surprised when Oprah, who admirably got many women out running, posted an "I Love Bread" video, sponsored by Weight Watchers (in which she is said to have an ownership stake). Noshing on bread is a sure prescription for *gaining* weight.

Hopefully, you can join me in the liberating knowledge that *miracle diets, products, and weight loss formulas simply do not work*. To some it may sound curious, to others self-apparent: if "diets" were successful at sustainably reducing weight, then people wouldn't need to obsessively follow them, and there would be no multibillion-dollar diet industry. Indeed, in the United States alone, $30 billion a year is spent on weight loss and diet programs. A diet plan that reliably *doesn't* succeed at helping people to maintain their weight loss presents the perfect business model: the customers are assured of returning for more treatment.

What are we to believe about all the nutrition and diet talk, anyway? As John P. A. Ioannidis, a professor of medicine and statistics at Stanford University, wrote, "Almost every single nutrient imaginable has peer reviewed publications associating it with almost any outcome. In this literature of epidemic proportions, associations, and flawed assumptions, with few high quality randomized trials, how many results are correct?"

What *does* work is far easier, healthier, and less expensive: eating healthfully and mindfully until you're full. You'll find that this "non-diet" is tastier, too—which is a clue to how it works. Over time, *no nutritional regimen can rely upon willpower*. Counting calories has one immediate problem: it causes you to think about, and sometimes obsess over, what you are eating throughout the day—which only draws attention to your hunger. (Try telling a smoker who is attempting to quit that he should spend the day thinking about cigarettes.) The glut of "diets" out there would enjoy a lot more success if, rather than prescribing austerity or enumerating calories and nutrients, they offered a delicious and filling meal.

Let's start by taking a look at what America is eating.

PYRAMIDS, PLATES, AND PRESIDENTIAL HOPE

The new *Dietary Guidelines for Americans* (DGA), released in early 2016, are an amendment to the original guidelines, issued forty years ago. By finally exonerating dietary fat and cholesterol, they are a step in the right direction, but are still a poor recipe for improving America's health. You might not have paid much attention to these guidelines, but millions of kids who eat school lunches are subject to them, military rations and SNAP (formerly known as food stamps) are tied to them, and their broad strokes trickle down into the public's perception of what's healthy.

The 2016 *Dietary Guidelines* emphasize, as they did in 1980, that fruits, veggies, beans/legumes, low-fat dairy, and whole grains form the foundation of a healthy diet. They correctly recommend that we reduce our sugar intake, and finally admit that, for healthy adults, *dietary* cholesterol and fat do not significantly elevate levels of *blood* cholesterol and fat, nor do they increase the risk of cardiovascular disease. And—finally, thankfully—eggs and coffee are off the "black" list.

It's true that this new, modified diet would, if followed carefully by the healthy and active 30 percent of the U.S. population that is insulin sensitive, result in maintenance of health. But the new guidelines still contain an abundance of carbohydrates, and again fail to address America's epidemic of obesity, type 2 diabetes, and prediabetes. Fat isn't even listed as a healthy nutrient, and the new guidelines ingrain the mistaken homily that dietary fat is a cause of obesity.

And despite a caution about sugar, the new guidelines allow diabetics ten added teaspoons per day—disregarding the immediate and long-term toxicity this presents. Imagine allowing a few cigarettes a day to emphysema or lung cancer patients. Indeed, it wasn't very long ago, before smoking was connected to cancer and lung disease, that doctors were endorsing cigarettes in television commercials. (Attend a medical conference, and at breaks watch the doctors head for the bagels, muffins, cookies, and sodas.)

President Kennedy vowed in 1962 that America would land a man on the moon before the end of the decade. Seven years later, that milestone was reached. By contrast, it has taken four decades for nutritionists and medical experts to *partly* understand the components of a healthy diet, then grudgingly (and incompletely) agree on how to describe it and promote it. Meanwhile, the United States ranks fiftieth in the world in health indicators such as obesity, diabetes, inactivity, and poor health. Based on this stark evidence, any scientist (or casual observer) can conclude that the U.S. guidelines *simply haven't worked.* It's not likely that the new, lightly amended version will do us much better.

How did this situation occur? To begin with, there's an inherent conflict of interest in the Department of Agriculture's dual mandates to advise the public about healthy food choices and to promote U.S. agricultural products (most of which end up in processed food). Looking further back, at human evolution, it was the agricultural revolution that domesticated *us,* not the other way around. When we turned from hunting and gathering to agriculture, we substituted a diverse menu of nutrient-rich foods for nutritionally depleted grains and seed oils, which tied us to cultivated land and crops.

I'm a member of the Nutrition Coalition, a nonprofit that advocates for sensible, science-based national nutrition policy. We launched a petition to Congress that has triggered funding for a thorough, independent scientific review of the current guidelines, with results due out in 2020. None too soon.

One small but positive development came with the demise, in 2015, of the Global Energy Balance Network, a "scientific" site funded by Coca-Cola that was designed to convince us that weight gain and loss was a matter of "energy balance." We now know this is not the case. After public disclosure of the network's funding streams to doctors and medical groups, Coke quietly and quickly closed the site.

In our hospital, we have thrown out the concept of "energy balance" altogether, and encourage patients to eat salads, veggies, eggs, meat, cheese, and fish—real food—to satiety. It's not their fault they have insulin resistance. It's because of the food that's heavily marketed and routinely placed in front of them. We initiated "Sugar Free JMC" (Jefferson Medical Center) in 2018, and are leading our state in getting sugar out of our health care environment.

THE MAGIC OF FAT

Contrary to what many assume, *healthy dietary fat does not make us fat*. Fat does not raise glucose or insulin levels. In fact, healthy fats have a remarkable ability to control weight—by satiating our hunger. When we eat foods in their natural (unprocessed) state, including healthy fats and protein, we become full sooner—and thereby stop eating. And we grow hungry later. Dietary fiber in veggies shares this hunger-satisfying effect, too.

But this hunger-satiating effect doesn't quite work when the fats travel with sugar and starch. When consumed with carbohydrates, dietary fat is metabolized and stored differently than when consumed in the absence of carbohydrates, and it affects our appetite in a different way. Bread and wraps, for instance, should be regarded as nothing more than vehicles to get the real food to your mouth. A better vehicle choice would be a utensil, or a large leafy green.

A study led by Christopher Ramsden revisited the diet-heart hypothesis and concluded that replacement of saturated fat in the diet with linoleic acid (a major ingredient in safflower oil and margarine) does not lower risk of death from coronary heart disease.

Healthy fats (those containing essential fatty acids and fat-soluble vitamins) are essential for maintaining a healthy body. Yet fat still doesn't appear as a food category on the government's widely disseminated "My Plate" nutritional health graphic.

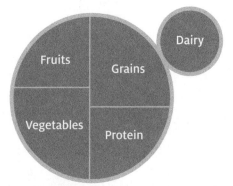

The "My Plate" health graphic replaced the "Food Pyramid,"
yet it still pushes grains (carbohydrates) and fruits (largely simple sugars).
The dairy they promote is low-fat. If you look at the foods typically
consumed in America, *more than 75 percent of this government-endorsed
meal plate can be composed of sugar and carbs.*

CHARTING YOUR PATH TO PERSONAL HEALTH

To determine whether you are glucose intolerant, you may want to check your post-meal glucose level on occasion, even if you're not diabetic. This can be done with a simple device called a glucometer, available in generic brands for less than $20. Eat a customary meal, then check your blood glucose level two hours later. It should be under 140 mg/dl. A higher figure indicates that you are not regulating glucose optimally.

As a prediabetic (but otherwise healthy) adult, if I ate a "healthy breakfast" consisting of a muffin, a big fruit bowl, sugar-sweetened yogurt, and juice—then skipped exercise and sat at a desk—my glucose level would easily go above 140 and stay there for some time. (The juice alone contains about 50 grams of carbohydrate.) When a diabetic person eats the same meal (as often happens, even in the hospital), they will consistently spike to over 200. This dangerously high post-meal glucose level might settle down and "reset" by the next morning (especially if insulin or other glucose-lowering meds are taken at night). But that imparts a false impression that all is well. Because many of these carb- and sugar-loaded foods are advertised as "natural" and may not contain "added sugar," most people don't realize that they are in fact consuming large amounts of sugar. Their "healthy breakfast" falls within the letter of the *Dietary Guidelines,* but is far from healthful.

SLAYING THE SWEET (BUT DANGEROUS) DRAGON

Diabetes and obesity are given lip service as life-threatening, yet they are more deadly and disabling than many cancers. It may sound hyperbolic (or for some, a tired refrain), but the *sugar-sweetened drinks and highly processed, high-carb foods are dragons that must be slayed.* This includes soft drinks, juices, sport drinks, sweetened milks, boost shakes, many types of smoothies, and most packaged yogurts—all of which are ubiquitous in our food system. If you are insulin resistant, the unique sugar in beer heads straight to the belly, too.

Okay, but how about those uber-fit mountain bikers and trail runners who drink gallons of craft beer?

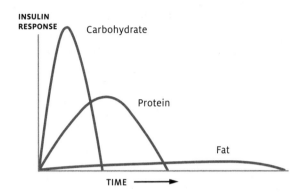

These curves show insulin release over time, by food type consumed, beginning right after eating a meal.

They can handle it—for a while. They are insulin sensitive, and likely young. Weight isn't normally a problem for elite athletes, because after years of frequent and high-intensity exercise (I'm picturing myself during college), they have become carbohydrate tolerant and insulin sensitive. They exercise hard and often, work up an appetite, and satisfy their hunger with a starch-heavy meal. Their insulin kicks in and does its job of storing sugar in the energy-hungry muscles, where it is ready for the next day's activity. Empty the tank, fill, and repeat.

Young Kenyan marathoners can live this way, too. But for how long? The human pancreas wasn't designed to handle the insulin demand from decades of processing 600 to 1,000 grams of carbs a day.

We do respond individually to sugar, just as we do to exercise. But as we age, we predictably begin to join the greater population—expanding in numbers and in waist circumference—that is carbohydrate intolerant and insulin resistant. For most of us (and virtually *all* of us at advancing ages), the excessive carbs we consume make a beeline for our stores of belly fat, piling onto whatever's already there.

WEIGHT LOSS STARTS IN THE KITCHEN

In something of a hopeful sign, people are just as active nowadays as they have been in the previous few decades. (This isn't quite true

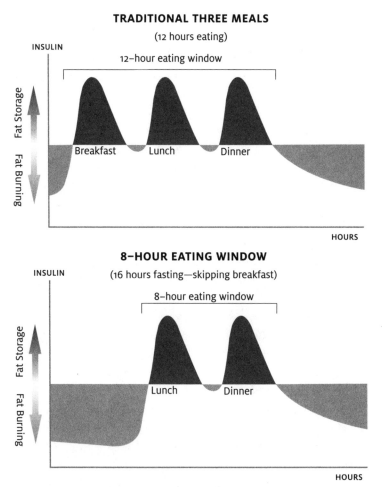

TRADITIONAL THREE MEALS
(12 hours eating)

INSULIN

12–hour eating window

Fat Storage

Fat Burning

Breakfast   Lunch   Dinner

HOURS

8–HOUR EATING WINDOW
(16 hours fasting—skipping breakfast)

INSULIN

8–hour eating window

Fat Storage

Fat Burning

Lunch   Dinner

HOURS

The shaded area above the midline in these graphs
represents the magnitude of fat that is stockpiled (= weight gain),
and the shaded area below the midline shows the burning of fat (= weight loss).
For fat to oxidize efficiently, insulin levels need to be low.
Thus frequent high-carb meals (and twenty-four-hour insulin injections, too)
sabotage the process of burning fat.

for children, unfortunately.) But exercise alone won't fix diabetes
or prediabetes. In fact, vigorous physical activity, which is mainly
a tool for building and maintaining muscle, is not associated with
significant weight loss. For most of us, the composition of what
we eat plays a far bigger role than exercise in maintaining body
weight. As the saying goes: ounces are lost in the gym, pounds are
lost in the kitchen and dining room.

EASE IS THE DISEASE

For millennia, humans have been on a constant search for sufficient food to eat. Harvard anthropologist Dan Lieberman describes this nutritional challenge, and how it has affected our evolution, in *The Story of the Human Body*. During the past century, and for the first time in human history, we have faced an unusual dilemma: food has become too abundant, cheap, convenient, easy to chew, and downright tasty for our own good. As a result, we eat large quantities of stuff that has lots of calories but tends to be of poor nutritional quality.

For our ancestors, gathering, hunting, or growing food was tedious. Processing and cooking it took time and effort. Now this scenario has been replaced by convenience and low cost, which have become the biggest obstacles to a healthy diet. It's too easy to dine at a restaurant or a fast-food joint, or grab inexpensive food to go. Many of us have abandoned the art and joy of preparing a healthful meal at home. As a fraction of total calories consumed, more than 62 percent of food in the American diet is highly processed. And less than 20 percent of the food America consumes requires cooking or preparation.

Eating well doesn't require shopping at health food stores or specialty markets. You can start with your chain supermarket and confine yourself, as best you can, to the display cases around the periphery. Focus on buying nonstarchy vegetables, meat, fish, nuts, olive oil, spices, lots of eggs, full-fat dairy, and unprocessed cheeses. If you aren't insulin resistant, whole fruit (pitted and nontropical, especially) and legumes can safely be added, along with small amounts of real, whole grains. Use these simple ingredients for virtually everything you prepare.

THE VIEW FROM LAST PLACE

Distressingly, most of America doesn't eat this way. My home state of West Virginia leads the nation in obesity, physical inactivity, and their metabolic consequences. Arkansas and Mississippi share with West Virginia an adult obesity rate of close to 40 percent.

Addressing this epidemic will require transformation of the way medical educators link the sciences of nutrition, biochemistry, and physiology to the clinical practice of primary care and community medicine. Hippocrates said, "Let food be thy medicine and medicine be thy food." But medical school curricula have almost totally neglected food and nutrition.

In response to this, in 2013 my colleagues and I developed a cooking, nutrition, and physical activity program for the West Virginia University School of Medicine called MedCHEFS—Medical Curriculum in Health, Exercise, and Food Science. Our goal is to teach medical students the scientific, clinical, and actionable aspects of healthy lifestyles, in a manner that will improve the health of our patients, our communities, and ourselves.

Armed with the concepts in this book, our medical students enter the kitchen, prepare and cook healthful (mostly low-carb) meals, then participate in sessions on fitness, proper body movement, and lifelong, joyful activity. By the end, they see the importance of establishing a collaborative relationship with their patients in order to prevent disease and to cultivate overall health. Medical and health decisions are made *with* the patient, not *for* the patient, prescribing health and restoration.

Some have questioned the relevance of learning about food and exercise in medical school. The response is simple: nearly every chronic disease is either driven or greatly affected by what we put in our mouths and what we do with our bodies. A program of disease prevention and healing, through modification of diet and lifestyle, is truly the best form of care we can offer.

The great news that accompanies all of this is that healthy eating, which comes in countless forms, is remarkably nonrestrictive. Healthful meals include fresh, hearty, rich foods with plenty of fat. Add butter (from grass-fed cows, preferably) to anything you want. Then go out and exert at a comfortable level, on a routine basis. There's no hurry. We are ready right now to begin dining sumptuously—for the rest of our healthy lives. *Bon appétit!*

DRILLS

The "exercises" in this chapter are presented as simple, sustainable dietary principles that attempt to answer the question "What should my family and I eat to be healthy?" The first, foundational exercise is straightforward: the next time you enter a distraction-crammed supermarket, shop with knowledge, awareness, and discipline. Make that *every* time you shop.

Dr. Mark's revised dietary guidelines for America
Try these simplified shopping, cooking, and eating guidelines for a period of one month.

- *Get rid of the sugar bowl,* and cut out added sugar entirely. Eliminate sugared drinks, including juice and sports drinks. (This step alone, if you are a significant sugar consumer, will boost your health noticeably and significantly.)
- *Upgrade all the components of your diet.* Include lots of healthy fats and quality protein—eggs, nuts, seeds, olive oil, avocados, whole fat dairy, cold-water fish, nonprocessed meats. Eat from a rainbow: colorful vegetables should be integral to every meal.
- *Go against the grains.* Eliminate processed foods and refined grains and flour products such as bread and pastries, especially if you're trying to reduce weight; learn your level of carbohydrate tolerance, and don't exceed it. (Check by looking in the mirror for a "muffin top" over your belt.) Avoid "food products," packaged meal replacements, and foods that list ingredients you can't pronounce. As Dr. Harry Lodge says, "Don't eat crap."
- *Remove all trans fats and vegetable seed oils* (corn, vegetable, canola, and safflower oils, and margarines), which are known to exacerbate inflammation. Go for real butter, coconut oil, avocado oil, and first-press olive oil. If the fat tastes good in its natural state then it likely is good. Avoid all foods labeled "diet," "low-fat,"

or "low-calorie." The fats in "low-fat" foods have almost certainly been replaced with carbs. Fat-soluble vitamins and minerals can't be utilized by the body without the fat itself.

- *Abandon all complicated, heavily prescriptive or overly restrictive diet regimens.* Don't go hungry! Eat until you are nearly full, not more.

That's how healthy eating works. The operative word is *simplicity*.

Some recipes I can't resist sharing

Here are my favorite go-to dishes, well suited to those of us with busy lives and affordable for most. The prep time for any of these, once the ingredients are gathered, should be no more than five minutes.

- *The stinky omelet.* That's what my kids affectionately call it. Take three farm-fresh eggs and add any meat, cheese, or veggie you have. Top it with homemade guacamole: salsa, salt, a little lime juice, and a mashed avocado.
- *Slow-cooked whatever meat is on sale.* Your local market often has a big hunk of pork shoulder, brisket, rump roast, or whole chicken at a sale price because it's a day past the sell-by date. That's fine, because you will cook it in a slow cooker for eight hours. Add a simple seasoning rub. Use the extra for meals and salads later in the week.
- *First-press olive oil on any leafy green.* This brings out a remarkable depth of flavor to most bitter greens, and facilitates vitamin and mineral absorption. It's no accident that cultures around the world add fat to vegetables. Simply pour some high-quality (dark green) olive oil over your uncooked greens, and add some salt. *Massage it in* with your hands for a couple of minutes. Top it off with high-quality balsamic vinegar (Kirkland brand, available at Costco and at a low cost, is a good one) and whatever else you like.
- *Bone broth.* This is magic for joints and fascia. From a butcher, get the bones (especially from grass-fed beef

or free-range chickens), including all the cartilage and marrow. Place in a crock pot with water, celery, carrots, an onion, and salt. Let stew for twenty-four hours.

- *Kale and walnut pesto.* This is a low-budget alternative to regular pesto. Mix together ½ cup of hard Italian cheese (Parmesan, pecorino Romano), ¼–½ cup of walnuts, ½ cup of olive oil, 2 cups of loosely packed kale, a clove of garlic, and salt. Mix in a food processor. Use this to top anything.
- *Micro bacon.* Use farmers' market bacon, if possible. In a microwave bacon pan, microwave for about a minute per slice, if thickly cut. Perfect every time, and no mess.

CHAPTER 11

Recovery *Is* the Training

*Once reduced to "the plod" it's only a matter of time before
injury, illness, or poor performance occurs. We've come to
understand this is a protective response of an exhausted body.*
—BRUCE FORDYCE,
nine-time Comrades Marathon champion

MYTH: *If we want to become stronger and healthier, we must
exert at the highest capacity we can tolerate.*

FACT: *Technically, it's only during recovery that we become
stronger and healthier. Adequate sleep, nutritious food, and
relaxed, comfortable movement are the most important
contributors to this process.*

Racing is optional. But rest and recovery after any vigorous activity is mandatory. Recovery is the time when your body repairs and strengthens, which doesn't happen while you are exerting. Recovery should not become a routine of rehabilitation and physical therapy.

The body has marvelous built-in mechanisms for adaptation, repair, and remodeling. When stresses are applied to the bones, tendons, and muscles, the body grows stronger as the repair work does its magic. But this presupposes the *right* amount of stress (also known as eustress), and also adequate time for the rebuilding process to occur.

The inflammation (and free radical production) in our muscles that follows mild stress is transitory and good—or mostly so. When tenderness or pain accompany inflammation, it is a signal to rest and protect ourselves. If instead we persist with high levels of physical and emotional stress, and a poor diet, we are setting our-selves up for *chronic* oxidative stress and inflammation. Chronic inflammation (literally meaning slow burning fire) is mostly invis-ible, can occur in any tissue or organ, and makes us vulnerable to disease and deterioration.

JUST SAY NO TO NSAIDS

Contrary to popular belief, nonsteroidal anti-inflammatory drugs (NSAIDs) such as ibuprofen and naproxen *don't* help with recov-ery, because they short-circuit the mild inflammation that is an integral part of the repair and rebuilding process. Cortisone injec-tions are worse: injections into or around an injured tissue may offer some pain relief, but they interrupt the repair and remodeling process.

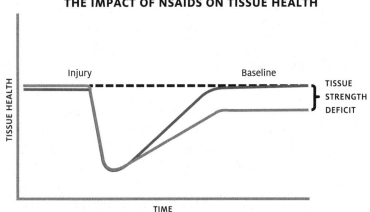

THE IMPACT OF NSAIDS ON TISSUE HEALTH

The body will always try to heal. Chronic usage of NSAIDs impacts the repair process and prevents the body from healing back to baseline tissue strength. This weaker, impaired tissue is now at a greater risk for reinjury.

THE HEART OF TRAINING

Many elite endurance athletes experience orthopedic overuse inju-ries such as plantar fasciitis, Achilles tendonitis, shin splints, and chondromalacia patella. But researchers are increasingly finding that *overtraining* and too much endurance racing may be more damaging to another key organ—the heart—than previously suspected. Sports cardiologists caution that cardiac overuse may be associated with *right heart* cardiac strain and failure, cardiac arrhythmia, accelerated coronary plaque formation, premature aging of the heart, myocardial fibrosis, plaque rupture, acute coronary thrombosis, and even sudden cardiac death.

One friend of mine, Boston Marathon director Dave McGillivray, exercised regularly until he had a wake-up call at age fifty-nine. Six months after the 2013 marathon—the year of the bombings—he was diagnosed with coronary heart disease. (The bombings had no doubt added to his overall stress.)

Following his diagnosis, he took what he had learned to heart, so to speak. He slowed down, cleaned up his diet, and lost thirty pounds. The day before the 2014 race he addressed the Sports Medicine Symposium of the American Medical Athletic Association (AMAA) as the picture of health, in body and spirit. He began by thanking the first responders who had treated the bomb victims the year before, then spoke about several of his physically fit running friends who had gone out for runs and hadn't made it home—felled not by improvised bombs but by heart attacks. "I spent a lifetime trying to be *fit,*" he said, "but I didn't spend time trying to be *healthy.*"

In the company of friends, Dave completed the race in the evening hours. Six months later, he qualified for and entered the grueling Ironman World Championship in Kona, Hawaii—the pinnacle of Ironman races. It was his first Ironman in twenty-five years, and he finished in a respectable 13 hours.

In addition to contributing to coronary inflammation, over-exercising (without sufficient recovery time) can leave scar tissue on the heart in the form of patchy cardiac fibrosis. This may afflict as many as 10 percent of today's serious marathon runners. The thick-walled left side of the heart can handle the stress, but the thin-walled right side seems better adapted to easy walking and jogging, not to daily hour-long high-tempo runs at the anaerobic threshold.

I've run many miles over the past thirty-five years, most of them at a comfortable pace. I feel fortunate that my echocardiogram and other markers of cardiac health check out normal.

HEART RATE VARIABILITY IS A GOOD THING

Recovery is often thought of in terms of tissue-specific work, such as foam rolling, gentle stretching, icing, contrast baths, or massage. But biological and hormonal recovery is just as important. The key indicators of this recovery are a lowered resting heart rate, healthy appetite, and improved mood and sleep patterns—along with a compelling desire to get out there and run again.

One emerging tool for assessing recovery and well-being is called *heart rate variability,* or HRV—a measure of the variation in the intervals between heartbeats. If your heart beats like a metronome, with intervals of identical length between each pulse, you have low HRV. A low HRV reading actually indicates poor recovery response and high sympathetic tone (or stress). If your heartbeat intervals vary, you have high HRV, which indicates more parasympathetic ("rest and digest") tone, better progression and responsiveness during recovery, and more stress reduction. Note that too much stress (and overtraining) tends to negatively affect your HRV, while quality sleep benefits it.

Until recently, measuring HRV required expensive monitoring devices found only in cardiac labs. But a good-quality Bluetooth heart rate monitor, paired with an inexpensive app such as Sweet Beat or Nature Beat, can now readily measure HRV. I use an app to measure my HRV several times a week, upon awakening, and the results seem to correspond well with my workload, sleep quality, level of recovery, and overall stress level. A low HRV reading (with more of a metronome-like beat) indicates that I should dampen the pace of my daily run to "slow jogging" level. That's not a problem. As counterintuitive as it may seem, I look forward to slow jogging as much as to running at a higher pace. (My dog likes the slower pace, too, for the added sniffing opportunities.) Recovery is what it's all about, and even after a ridiculously slow run I always feel better.

DREAM THROUGH YOUR RECOVERY

One of the most important recovery drills couldn't be more straightforward: sleep. The benefits of sleep to mental function, neurocognition, and hormonal restoration are well known, even if the mechanisms by which they restore us are not entirely understood. We could reasonably refer to it as "sleep doping," for its remarkably beneficial effects. If sleep was not necessary, it would be evolution's greatest mistake.

Sleep doesn't come easily for many of us. Three-quarters of Americans are walking around with a sleep deficit. In the absence of sound, restorative sleep, our appetite increases, insulin resistance increases, growth hormone is suppressed, tissue repair is inhibited, and mood is altered.

How do you feel? Tired? Uninspired? In a sour mood? If so, going to bed earlier and maintaining good sleep habits may be the single most important health advice I can offer.

Sleep is divided into REM (rapid eye movement) sleep and NREM (the nonrapid kind). NREM is further divided into stages N1, N2, and N3. Slow wave sleep, N3, is the deepest and longest. REM comprises 20 percent of a night's sleep, and is when most of our dreaming and rebuilding occurs, and when the powerful recovery hormones testosterone and estrogen are released.

We progress consecutively through all four stages in approximately ninety-minute cycles. Most of us need five to six full sleep cycles each night. If you have a sleep shortfall for a day or so, you can make up for much of it with a soundly restful night or two (during the weekend, for instance). Even a nap can pick up a lost cycle.

A hormone called melatonin promotes sleep. But at night, artificial light has the opposite effect, by throwing the circadian rhythm—the body's biological clock—out of whack. Blue light wavelengths inhibit the release of melatonin more than other colors, and are especially disruptive of sleep.

It's best to not view digital screens, including smartphones, for at least an hour before bedtime. If you have to use a screen at night, you might try a free app called f.lux, for your computer, or Night Shift for your smartphone. They automatically transition your screen to a more amber light spectrum after sunset.

Another powerful regulator of sleep-wake cycles is the morning sun. A few extra minutes in the morning to run, walk the dog, or simply walk to (or park farther from) the office can do wonders for your daily wakefulness and the quality of your sleep.

Growth hormone (GH) is another hormonal recovery friend, and is secreted during the N3, slow wave sleep phase. (Waking a child from this stage is nearly impossible.) The duration of the N3 cycle decreases with age, partly explaining why we recover differently at age fifty than at twenty-five. Fragmented and foreshortened sleep causes the levels of blood sugar and cortisol to rise, curtailing the restorative functions and healthy healing of the body. Sleep apnea commonly travels with obesity and metabolic syndrome, and circumvents the important N3 sleep phase. This contributes to a vicious cycle of more physiologic stress and less recovery, resulting in a greater incidence of high blood pressure, heart disease, diabetes—and auto accidents.

EATING AFTER EXERCISE

During exercise, insulin-independent pathways for glucose utilization and disposal are activated in the muscles. In other words, the muscles and liver are more carbohydrate tolerant during exercise, and for up to an hour after a workout. This means that even if you are insulin resistant, there is a small window for a bit of what is called "carb backloading," and you may be able to consume *some* quality carbohydrates. You must earn your carbs!

The fastest way to recover from more intense workouts and races is to eat a healthy meal within the next hour. Recommended post-activity nutrition depends on your metabolism, muscle mass, genes, and goals. If you simply want to run for general health and fitness, without a specific goal of fat loss or diabetes reversal, then include some healthy whole food carbs with your fat and protein. The carbohydrates will elevate your blood sugar slightly, signaling the pancreas to release insulin. This drives the amino acids (protein building blocks) and essential fatty acids from the food and into the muscle cells, hastening healing and growth. The healthy low-carb food is your foundation, and the modest amount of carbs (only after exertion) act as a supplemental fuel refill for the tissues. Following a hot summer run, a side of fresh melon with some salt does wonders for me. Individual results will vary, so experiment!

Your goal should be to use fat as your primary fuel throughout the day. Have an omelet with some veggies, or a bunless burger in a leafy wrap. Athletes trying to reverse type 2 diabetes or obesity may want to learn about and test-run a ketogenic diet, which consists of quality, natural fats, adequate protein, and very few carbs. One eats to satiety, not in excess. This diet enlists ketone bodies—a breakdown product of fat metabolism—as a source of fuel for the brain and muscles. Full discussion of the science of a well formulated ketogenic diet is beyond the scope of this book. (See *The Art and Science of Low Carbohydrate Performance,* by Drs. Jeff Volek and Stephen Phinney.)

As part of your recovery, don't forget hydration. Follow your thirst. If you don't fully trust that, check your urine: the color of light beer is good. Darker than that (e.g., Guinness)—not so good. Add a squirt of lemon or lime to your water, for flavor. And before a summer run, drink some water with a small amount of dissolved sodium to help super-hydrate your cells. You'll be internally stashing an extra water bottle, in effect. For active, healthy people who are not salt sensitive, 3 to 5 grams of total sodium per day is the optimal healthy range—despite conventional wisdom suggesting salt's danger.

SLOW JOGGING AS A CURE FOR RUNNING

Another method of "active recovery" is slow jogging, especially good when the fascia is sticky and mildly inflamed and the muscles are restricted and sore.

I was honored to have Dr. Hiroaki Tanaka, a professor at Fukuoka University (see his book *Slow Jogging: Lose Weight, Stay Healthy, and Have Fun with Science-Based Natural Running*) participate in two of my Healthy Running courses. He calls his method of easy, relaxed jogging "*niko niko* running," or running with a smile, and it has become popular in Japan.

How to do it? Think about mastering the art of landing softly. Then begin slowly. Really slowly. Gently hop up and down a few times as if jumping rope, and land with softness and spring. Jog in place, then move a bit forward and backward. Breathe slowly and fill the belly. As best you can, move your body through its full range of motion.

One appealing feature of slow jogging is that you can do it anywhere—in the mall, at airports, and in the workplace. Running hard and fast comes later. Dr. Tanaka's program led him to a 2:38 marathon at age fifty.

AVOID THE BLACK HOLE OF TRAINING

Recovery is about taking time to manage your training and exertion level. If you try to maintain a fast pace every time you exercise—too fast to tap into your storage tanks of fat, yet not exactly sprinting or exerting anaerobically—you're training in what Dr. Stephen Seiler calls the "black hole of training." In the hybrid car analogy, you can detect this black hole when you *believe* you are cruising along efficiently, but then *see* that the MPG meter reads 15, instead of your estimated 99. You are in gas-guzzling (sugar) mode, which is not sustainable for long periods. You won't boost aerobic development.

Most athletes, from beginners to elites, spend too much of their training time in this gas-guzzling, high-end aerobic zone, and it ends up inhibiting their performance, with toxic effects. It's not a coincidence that marathoner Ryan Hall trained like a beast—above a level that his body could sustain—and then retired at thirty-three. Many athletes plateau at a level well below what they might have reached had they trained aerobically, at a slower pace.

That's where the adaptation curve comes in.

A plateau can be described as *level high ground*. Many of us never reach it. If too little recovery time is allowed, the body doesn't fully recover. That's overtraining. Repeatedly, I see proponents of the "no pain, no gain" approach who simply aren't able to maintain a high level of performance. As Arthur Lydiard said, "Train, don't strain." He understood and respected *hormesis*, or eustress: carefully dosed levels of stress, combined with rest, result in growth and success.

Now, at age fifty-one, I realize that my days of improving performance are likely over. In order not to lose ground, I look for the

THE ADAPTATION CURVE

- When you subject your body to a training workout, your fitness level temporarily decreases
- During the subsequent recovery period your fitness level will rebound beyond the previous fitness level
- This is called Super-Compensation

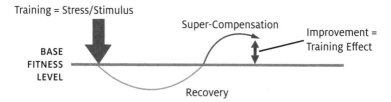

There's an old coaches' principle: *training success = moderate stress + adequate rest*. With any moderate or strenuous activity, fatigue eventually occurs and performance declines. That's followed by an adaptation/recovery phase in which super-compensation occurs, establishing a slightly higher platform of performance for the next period of exertion.

sweet spot of training: the point at which the load applied doesn't exceed my body's capacity to adapt. Frank Shorter said that the harder he trained with speed, the more he needed to recover with the gentle slow stuff.

In our busy lives, recovery may be difficult, but it's nonnegotiable.

DAILY RECOVERY VERSUS RACE RECOVERY

When planning your race or your workout session, think ahead to the all-important recovery phase and set an internal detector: if you feel you are having an exceptional, "breakthrough" race or training run, it can be a red flag. With unusual speed and strength comes a mild state of euphoria and a peak in adrenaline—which most of us read as a sign to *push harder*. Often as not, however, this is a warning sign that you are overtraining and at risk of throwing your recovery cycle out of synch, extending the time needed for recovery. You can't hurry a hen in her laying of eggs: you can only lay so many, and in certain seasons.

Seek a *high plateau*, not a *peak*. Find the pace at which you'll lay the maximum number of quality eggs over an extended period of time. Simply stated, any recovery activity—whether a walk, jog, massage, swim, or meditation—should make us feel better after the activity than we did before. We don't need to add stress to an already busy life.

IF IT DOESN'T FEEL GOOD, DON'T DO IT

Logically, my long barefoot runs on paved roads should be stressful to the bones and joints (not to mention the skin on the soles of my feet). But my body has adapted to years of minimal and barefoot running, which has made my feet essentially bulletproof. The muscles are thick and the bones dense from the constant loading and recovery.

The late running doctor and author George Sheehan often wrote that "we're all an experiment of one." Humans are all built much the same, though each of us responds to training, and to

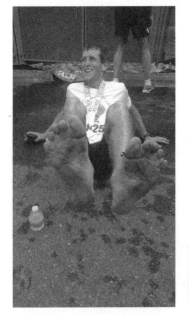

My feet after a 20K run on pavement

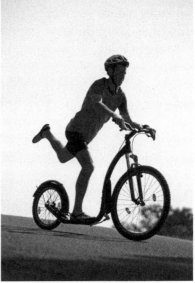

Recovery—on the Kickbike

recovery, a bit differently. Regardless of how we respond, there is one simple gauge that we can rely on: if we wake up with a spring in our step and a desire to run, then we are recovered. There's no shortcut or "hack" to getting there. The most thorough, endurance-enhancing recovery happens naturally and slowly, following moderate, healthful stress. If your workouts are less brutal, your enjoyment will be greater and your recovery faster and easier. And your performance will improve. A win-win-win.

DRILLS

An unconventional treat for your feet

One unusual (and counterintuitive) recovery drill is to take off your shoes and run barefoot on pavement: this forces you to step gently and to slow down. Bare feet connecting with smooth pavement triggers the two hundred thousand proprioceptive nerve endings in the feet to "reset" the mechanoreceptors in the fascia and muscles. It's what I call "active recovery." No need for NSAIDs, nutritional supplements, a cold river, or a room full of devices.

I discovered this in 2011 after running the Boston Marathon, which has lots of downhills. The day after the race I was stiff and sore, as expected, and the most comfortable option would have been to transfer myself from bed to lounge chair to plane. But the morning was beautifully sunny and I desperately wanted to get outside. The thought of putting on my shoes was not a happy one, so I set off slowly down Commonwealth Avenue in my bare feet. (I had earlier experienced some of the mysterious benefits of barefoot running.) After an hour of very gentle running and movement, I felt rejuvenated, ready for playful activity.

Try this, and see where it takes you.

Recover from running by sprinting

This sounds counterintuitive, too, but try finishing your run by opening up your stride and doing some short sprints (and throw in some skips and relaxed running form drills). You'll end up fully mobile and symmetric, because sprints work like dynamic stretching and set you up for better recovery. So—fly a little at the end of your run! If you finish an exercise session in a tight position, you'll start the next day in a tight, locked, compromised position.

Sleep loose

One of the most important recovery drills couldn't be easier: sleep. At least two hours before bed, don't eat sugar, turn off digital screens, find a cool, quiet place, and retire early (so that you don't need an alarm to wake up). Most of us sleep with our mouths wide open, which is not optimally healthful because we tend to draw in shallow breaths with the upper rib cage. I've found that a nasal dilator (such as Nasal Turbine) facilitates nose breathing during sleep, which boosts the parasympathetic system by allowing more diaphragmatic breathing. Or try placing a strip of tape over your mouth at night.

And get to know your baseline heart rate variability (HRV), and respect that number. Upon awakening, do some slow, deep nasal breathing, then check your HRV reading. This should be a beacon to your level of effort for that day, with a high HRV meaning that it's okay to train today.

Water
Soaking in water is magical. Some like it hot, and some like it cold. I'm a skinny old guy, and the mere thought of jumping into cold water is stress-inducing. I have a small hot tub on the back porch, and I relax and do gentle mobilization in it at the end of the day. Water supports and massages the body in ways that nothing else can.

Foam rolling
Gentle fascia mobilization with foam rollers helps keep the fascia and muscles supple. Experiment with your tight spots—generally the hip flexors, quads, calves, and thoracic spine. Rolling should never be rushed or rough. Using different shapes and sizes of tubes, or even a lacrosse ball, roll along the belly of the muscle and into the grooves separating the muscles. Pause over a spot occasionally, take a deep abdominal breath, and flex and extend the joint. This is my five-minute morning routine of gentle tissue flossing. I follow that with some easy hip movement.

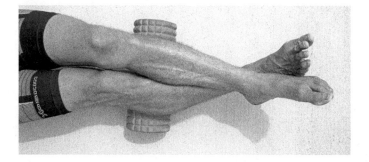

Compression

The soleus muscle—the calf—is referred to as the "second heart," because of its ability to activate blood and lymphatic fluid return to the heart, mostly through the simple act of walking. If you sit for extended periods in a car or airplane, or at a desk, or have been confined to a bed (which is best avoided, even in hospitals), then compression socks can help. They aren't substitutes for walking and moving, however. It's always best to move and recover actively. Walk it off. But if you can't, compress.

The market is flooded with compression products—in every color imaginable, for every part of the body. The effects of gravity and distance from the heart mean that the lower extremities are the most important to compress, and can aid in reducing swelling and discomfort from long periods of sitting or standing. Make sure you get medical-grade products.

The mind

Recovery of the mind is essential. If you have been training hard and enter an event, the adrenaline high will be followed, predictably, by a letdown. Anticipate this and give your mind some rest and flexibility, in whatever way works best and fits your schedule. Take breaks from the running regimen.

CHAPTER 12

Running a Marathon

It's very hard in the beginning to understand that the whole idea is not to beat the other runners. Eventually you learn that the competition is against the little voice inside you that wants to quit.

—GEORGE SHEEHAN, M.D.

Everyone should run one marathon. The rest is optional.

—MEB KEFLEZIGHI

MYTH: *Races are all about winning, or improving your race time.*

FACT: *Races should be about setting a goal and achieving it, and about joy, sharing, and health.*

MYTH: *To run your best time, you must run "hard."*

FACT: *Running your best is all about relaxing and harnessing the inherent efficiency of the human body.*

For some it can be tedious to exercise and train alone, day after day. As humans, we seek challenging experiences, and we desire to engage with others—to play, to strive, to get in the game—because it's fun. Without a challenge, there is no growth. So we enter a race.

As the number of running race entrants has grown, so have the stakes. Events have become more competitive. Times have improved. Distances have lengthened. Obstacles and challenges (such as Death Valley, or mountain passes) have been introduced. Almost inadvertently, an entire subculture has arisen around the ultra-marathon and Ironman circuits, with entrants racing frequently and for prize money. In 1965, the Boston Marathon had fewer than three hundred entrants. By 2017, thirty thousand runners took to the course—fifty thousand ran in the New York Marathon the same year. Many thousands more never reach the ever-tightening qualifying standards.

As your strength, endurance, and joy increase (because of the principles you've applied from this book), it's natural that you'll feel ready to enter a race. But run in a race only if you are well prepared and if you are confident that it will bring you joy. Too often, obsessive runners harm themselves by not sufficiently slowing down and preparing for longer distances. They are tearing themselves down, rather than building health.

ONE STEP AFTER ANOTHER

Like many, I have regarded the marathon as a lifetime goal, and feel privileged as a representative of the U.S. Air Force to have run twenty-five Marine Corps Marathons, fourteen Air Force Marathons, and twenty-four Boston Marathons. I'm still learning, and I love to share what I've learned with others.

The biggest milestone en route to running a marathon comes when you are able to run three miles comfortably. That first three miles—5K—will happen only when you have established a foundation of health and fitness. Once you can run a 5K race, you can run a 10K.

Running a marathon successfully, on the other hand, involves science, overall health, faith in yourself, smart training, discipline, restraint, creativity, and a small load of luck. So, what do you get in return for that investment of time and energy? The marathon distance offers little or no health advantage over shorter races, such as the half marathon. (Over the 26.2 miles of a marathon, the runner takes more than fifty thousand punishing steps, after all.) But entering a marathon is an empowering undertaking. And simply finishing conveys confidence into other parts of one's life. And if you can run a marathon, chances are that you can readily step out and run shorter distances.

I'd like to share with you the strategies that you can use to build and maximize your level of performance as marathon race time gets closer. You can apply this to a half-marathon event as well.

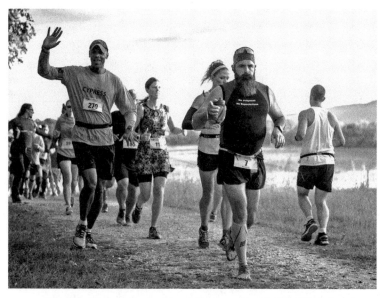

Friends set out on the Freedom's Run marathon in West Virginia.

DON'T EAT AND RUN . . .

Running a marathon for me, at age fifty-one, entails cranking out 6:45 miles—which admittedly is faster than the training speed dictated by my maximum aerobic heart rate. Four to six weeks before a race, I'll do some six- to ten-mile runs at this quicker, marathon pace, just to feel the coordination of movements needed and to dial in the sensation of relaxing at a faster speed.

Most of the time, I do what I call metabolic training. I teach my body to maximize its aerobic fitness (and to burn fat) by *not eating* before or during my long runs. When fasted, the active body adapts to its (foodless) environment. If sugar is readily accessible (following a high-carb meal, for instance), then the body doesn't bother switching to fat-burning mode. If you eat carbs, you'll end up burning carbs (at least some of them). But if you eat fats (or don't eat at all), you'll burn more fats—if, that is, you haven't jacked up your insulin response by eating carbs. *Insulin inhibits the body's utilization of fats as fuel.* This is critical to understand.

Long runs in a fasted state—as much as two hours at an easy to moderate pace—drain the slow-twitch ("red," oxidative, aerobic) fibers of their glycogen, and force more capillarization of the fast-twitch (mixed aerobic/anaerobic, largely "white") fibers. This shifts the fast-twitch muscles into a more aerobic (oxidative) state. In essence, when you run before eating you are adapting your body to function better in a carbohydrate-depleted state, by teaching it to draw on the stores of energy that are the most abundant and efficient—the fat. You're instructing your muscles' slow-twitch fibers (and even the fast-twitch oxidative fibers) to generate more fat-fueled energy.

You may want to try some fasted long runs before your next marathon. Race day itself will be different, because you'll be going for outright performance, not creating *adaptations* for performance.

Remember that the sweet spot for working out is thirty to sixty minutes of movement, most days of the week. As you ramp up to a marathon or half marathon, extending this to two or three hours, one day a week, will get you to the start line healthy and hungry to run.

THREE DAYS PRIOR

Three days before a marathon, fill your glycogen stores by resting and eating fat, protein, and topping off with some healthy carbohydrates. Don't overeat, and don't "load." You can store only so much. Fat is the primary fuel, but you might as well fill the sugar tank, too.

And sleep. Follow your usual routine, and avoid being on your feet all day. Do some relaxed running—jog slowly a few miles. Relaxation takes precedence over training. You may be traveling the day before a race anyway. It's best not to fill your head with whatever else you might have done to maximize your training and readiness. If you make it to the starting line in good health, injury-free, and confident in your preparations, you're almost to the finish line.

THE NIGHT BEFORE . . .

Psychological preparation is as important as physical fitness. The race day checklist should include a *mental* plan for dealing with adverse conditions, because it is completely normal to have bad patches. (With relaxation and a reset when you are struggling, you can usually emerge and shake it off.) Anticipate this by rehearsing complete relaxation from the top down—eyes, jaw, shoulders, arms, legs.

Self-confidence is critical. Visualize all the miles you have *already* run. Place yourself in the frame of mind that *you have completed the real work.* The race is just the final touch, the final lap, the fun part.

Four-time Olympic Trials qualifier Josh Cox offered me a great tip for putting your mind at ease the night before a race: on the floor, lay out your outfit and gear—everything that you'll wear or use the next day—in the shape of an "invisible man." On race day, scrambling to find your bib number, socks, favorite hat, or other items only adds stress. Then get some sleep! At a talk two days before the 2016 Air Force Marathon, I mentioned the "invisible man." The next day, a runner came up to me with a smile and a new pair of running shoes. She said she went home after the talk, laid out her gear, and realized she had forgotten her shoes.

RACE DAY MORNING

Don't sabotage your performance by consuming a large, carbohydrate-heavy breakfast, which would elevate your insulin levels and hijack the ability to burn fat. Have a light breakfast of fat, protein, and a small amount of carbs, along with your morning coffee if you're a coffee drinker. For me, this amounts to a banana with some almond butter a couple of hours before the start, and a shake of low-carb UCAN about an hour prior. I like a product called VESPA, too, which supports fat metabolism.

THE START . . . AND THE EARLY MILES

To sum up the best mind-set to adopt for a race of *any* distance, it's: *relax*. Don't start a race too fast. Your objective, from the starting gun, should be to dial in the proper balance between your fat and sugar fuels, such that you're optimally efficient for the duration of the race. Going too hard early on will deplete the sugar stores—the gas tank—and shunt too much blood to working muscles. You need to tap into your reservoir of fat (electricity), using the same metabolism that allows a bird to migrate thousands of miles without an aid station. It's all about pace. You're migrating.

FARTHER ALONG . . . ENERGY MONITORING

For a marathon, your sugar stores of blood glucose (less than 20 kcal), liver glycogen (300–500 kcal), and muscle glycogen (1000–1500 kcal) provide you with only about half the needed energy to get you the full distance. This is why it is essential to draw as much energy as possible from your own body fat. It's best to rely on "electricity" and conserve "gas" early in the race. Operate in hybrid mode, and cruise on the electricity as much as you can.

Carry a few glucose gels with you at the start. If you can take in a bit of glucose along the way, then you can permit yourself to run a bit more in gas mode if called upon. If you're running too fast or if the temperature is high, however, your blood migrates to the skin to help with cooling—which diverts blood from the gut, so nothing digests. If you have remained in hybrid, sugar/fat mode in the early stages, you can add small quantities of glucose along the way. After the start, a gel every sixty minutes can usually be digested and helps top off the tank. This helps maintain mental energy, too: studies have shown that even swishing a sports drink in your mouth (and not ingesting any) delays exhaustion.

If you take gels, you can drink water (according to your thirst) and avoid the energy drinks, which have an unpredictable glucose content. (The Marine Corps Marathon, for example, has twelve water points and four food stations.) But don't drink too much water, as it can lead to a dangerous condition called hyponatremia.

Calorie-free electrolytes like UCAN Hydrate are great to add to water and easy to carry. You might also want to study the tips on pages 198–199 for running in the heat, when hydration needs increase.

HYBRID MODE VIGOR

So, how do you know when you are running in your best hybrid mode? That's tricky to say, because it's difficult to sense the subtle but important aerobic threshold as readily as the more profound anaerobic (or lactate) threshold, discussed in chapter 7. A slight increase from your optimal pace may cause you to exceed the aerobic threshold, and quietly switch you from hybrid mode to all gas. The effects will be felt miles later, when your energy crashes.

If you're tempted to apply some speed early on, I have one recommendation: *don't*. Instead, relax and maintain a comfortable effort and pace (though your speed may change). You should feel comfortable in the early stages. It's a marathon, after all.

I try to belly breathe, by filling the lower reaches of the lungs where more complete oxygen exchange occurs. If I'm taking an in-breath and out-breath (one cycle) for every five steps, then I'm in sustainable hybrid mode. If I'm breathing faster, then I'm burning mostly gas—glucose—as fuel. Notice the breathing efforts of those around you. Many will be breathing rapidly, and they are the ones likely to suffer after the halfway point. If you use a heart rate monitor in training, consider wearing it during the event.

TECHNIQUE AND STRATEGY

Avoid the tendency to overstride, and go smoothly and easily on the downhill stretches (where you can damage your quads). Allow gravity to assist you. And if it's windy, get behind a group and slipstream—it will save physical and mental energy. Allow your legs to relax and extend behind you. Your core is strong and solid, your legs are the springs.

In 2002, I ran alongside legendary three-time Boston women's

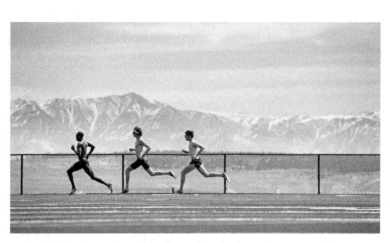

When you relax and let the springs do the work—you can fly!

winner Uta Pippig of Germany until she dropped me at Cleveland Circle, Mile 22. The crowds loved Uta, and the cheering and noise swelled as she approached. She smiled the whole way, and I wonder if this was how she cued herself to relax, as she fed off the crowd's energy, present in the moment. You could barely hear her footfalls—she ran *over* the road, not *into* it. Her posture was tall, her arms relaxed, and she efficiently used and conserved energy.

Uta ran 2:28 that day, a strong fourth place, and I finished a few strides behind her in 2:29. She exemplified how our brains govern our effort: when we are positive-minded, energy naturally flows through the body.

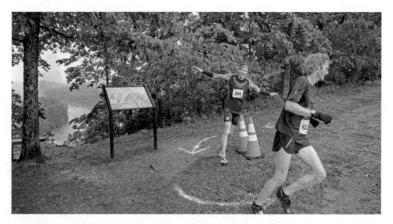

Smiling and flying at the Harper's Ferry Half Marathon

THE LAST FEW MILES

You have hopefully saved some energy for the later stages of the race, which is where things get tough and life can seem miserable. Fatigue will set in, your springs will lose bounce, and your heart rate will rise. At this point, you can't afford to think about how far you have to go or about how relieved you'll feel later, or if you're going to hit the wall and slow down.

You'll spend the last three to four miles mostly in gas (sugar-burning) mode as you try to maintain speed. Your breathing rate will elevate until you're getting only four, or sometimes three, steps per breath cycle. This is fine. You've conserved gas. Stay relaxed, and speed up only when you can "smell the barn," which typically occurs around Mile 23. (In Boston, that's when you see the Citgo sign.)

From training, you have built and enhanced your running form. But your form will begin to "drift" as you fatigue. You'll become sloppier. Simply remember to land softly (especially on the downhills) and think:

- Don't overstride.
- Harness elastic recoil.
- Keep posture erect: run tall.
- Face forward and look ahead.
- Maintain good hip extension.
- Relax arms, like chicken wings.
- Run *over* the ground, not *into* the ground.
- Find and maintain rhythm.
- Relax your lower jaw.

Try to avoid movements that are painful—even though *all* movement by now may feel uncomfortable. Make adjustments to your style. Play around, while maintaining your rhythm and spring. Distractions abound on the sidelines, but for you there are no distractions. Just peace in the moment. Relax.

A decline in blood glucose can trigger a sense of doom—so take in a few calories. And when you hit Mile 21, think of it not as five miles to go, but four and change. Mile 22 is three and change.

Compartmentalize each mile by running a single mile at a time, counting down the mile markers. Have faith in your training and race plan. Smile and take a moment to enjoy the crowds, if an urban race, or the peaceful setting if in the countryside.

MANAGING YOUR MIND

The best marathoner in the world, Eliud Kipchoge, says, "A smile is what actually ignites my mind to forget about the pain. That's the beauty of a smile."

The most important organ used in running is the brain—your mission control. Competitive runners learn how to interpret and respond to the signals that the body sends to their brains. The sensation that you have reached your capacity for further effort— the moment when your brain says *You're done*—generally occurs when you have utilized only about 60 percent of your capacity. The brain is going to protect you from harm, and is designed with a self-limiting governor. But it is also designed with work-arounds that allow you to turn off the initial messages and tap into another level of reserves. You can talk back to your brain and tell it that you need and want to continue.

Nonetheless, the brain, which likes homeostasis, will resist your persistence (*Twenty-six miles? You gotta be kidding . . .*), and it will urge you to slow down or stop. It will read your physical state as one of serious peril. That's when "sympathetic" stress kicks in and your level of cortisol elevates—which is good for sprinting from a wild animal but not for marathon-style hunting.

So, assuming you are medically healthy, you'll need to outwit your brain.

How to do that?

Work around the bad patches by cultivating (and remaining in) the parasympathetic, stress-free zone. Seek out a calm, stable zone for your mind. Alter your stride. Sing a song. Slow the breathing. Again, relax.

You made it!

SHORT IS BEAUTIFUL

Now, after all this discussion about running a marathon, I'm going to admit something that may surprise you: competing in marathons isn't always healthy for us. If the pre-race training is relaxed, aerobic, and fun, the occasional marathon can be a worthy challenge. But the level of effort needed for racing competitively over that distance should be tapped into infrequently. I recommend running no more than two or three marathons a year. A total of one is perfectly fine for a lifetime.

You can't hurry a chicken laying quality eggs: there is a season for it, and an interval between events, and there are no shortcuts or hacks. When runners train too hard and race too frequently, they end up in a chronic state of managing recovery debt. Their bodies don't catch up.

In terms of health, the half marathon is safer than a marathon because there is less chance of injury from repetitive stress. Nearly two million runners entered half marathons in 2017—almost four times the number that entered and finished marathons. (More women than men raced in events of *every* distance.)

The 5K and 10K runs are all-gas, mostly sugar-burning events. A glycogen-conserving strategy isn't needed for races of less than an hour, as long as you've filled your tank with a healthy meal the night before. But when runners who are in "great 10K shape" try to run a marathon in all-gas mode, they tend to crash when their glycogen stores run out.

If you are hesitant about running a marathon, yet it still seems to be drawing you, then run it for someone, or for a cause. I coached the Leukemia & Lymphoma Society Team in Training in Denver for several years. My wife, Roberta, a pediatrician, ran her first marathon in Cozumel after committing to this cause.

WHERE A MARATHON TAKES US

Perhaps the best reason to run a marathon is that it can act as a waypoint in overcoming what for most of us are daunting obstacles: inertia, distraction, and busy-ness. I have an insanely hectic

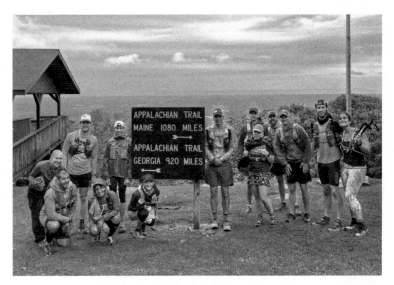

The power of the group makes us stronger.

life, and find myself rationalizing that there are more productive ways to spend my time than to run through the woods or enter a race. But once I've dropped everything, torn myself away, and am out running on the trail or road, I am *always* thankful.

The next time you are running, ask yourself: "Do I regret coming out?" Time spent on the road or on trails is a modest price to pay for the health and well-being you gain.

Uncertainty abounds every time I queue up at the starting line. But I learn something new each race. Mainly, I've learned that significant challenges, such as marathons, are what make us human, and make us better fathers, mothers, and friends.

DRILLS

In the appendix, page 314, please see the 16-week Marathon Plan (from the *Military Times*), and the links to my training info in Dr. Mark's Desk, which is linked in the book's web portal, runforyour lifebook.com. These plans and schedules aren't rigid requirements, even if you're planning to run a marathon. They are meant to help gauge whether you are on the right track to the starting line. The race itself is the final lap.

A note on racing in the heat

Race conditions such as heat or humidity can make a mockery of weeks, if not months, of sustained training.

Forty-eight hours before the 2012 Boston Marathon, the race committee alerted the participants that the race temperature would be in the "red zone" and prudently warned that although hydration is important, overhydration is dangerous.

The Boston course temps reached into the nineties. Race officials treated nearly 2,100 cramping and weary runners in three air-conditioned medical tents stationed along the course and at the

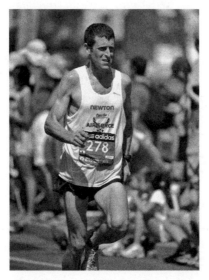

Meet the heat. Boston Marathon, 2012.

finish line. More than 150 were sent to hospitals. Many of the elite runners didn't finish.

Heat is a powerful brake. I played it safe and finished nine minutes slower than my time the previous year (but came away with fourth in the forty-five-to-forty-nine age group). More important, I avoided the medical tent by following good racing practices.

Too often, runners mistakenly believe that drinking a copious amount of water will lower the body's core temperature. But overdrinking won't cool you down. Cooling comes primarily from an evaporative effect. I repeatedly cooled myself by pouring water over my head and body. Thankfully, the humidity was low enough for this to work—the water actually evaporated.

Conventional wisdom is that the body will somehow dry up if we lose fluid. But "dehydration"—a nonclinical term with no real definition—is normal to a degree. Typically, the best runners finish marathons in a "dehydrated" state, with core temperatures above baseline. But they are not ill, just appropriately warm and tired and in need of some recovery. An ingrained human response of "I am hot and must drink more" is slowly being replaced with "I am thirsty, so I should drink." Not surprisingly, heatstroke occurs more frequently in *shorter* events, when the body's engine is working at max output.

Here are a few marathon cooling strategies—inspired, you might say, by our own human evolution:

- If warm conditions are predicted, try to preacclimate. Emerging from a winter of running, especially, the body needs to reengage the sweat mechanisms. Simply overdress for your training runs. In seven to fourteen days of acclimation, you will increase plasma volume, lower heart rate during exercise, decrease sodium concentrations in sweat, increase the sweating rate, and enhance blood delivery to the skin.
- Drape an ice-cold towel or splash cold water over yourself before the race, which will let you take on more thermal load. Don't warm up beforehand. Have an electrolyte popsicle.
- Keep the body wet, for evaporative cooling. Grab water on the run and pour it over you. Use sunscreen sparingly

(only on key areas, such as your nose) because it beads the sweat and water, and that water rolls off without evaporating. The evaporation of water on the surface of your skin is what cools you.

- Seek out and move toward the shady parts of the route, even if it means a few added steps. Radiant heat is direct thermal gain from the sun.
- Avoid running in a tight pack. Get some air around you and avoid absorbing the heat generated by a crowd.
- Drink when you are thirsty. You may want to carry a bottle and take sips, which is preferable to chugging water at an aid station. You *will* lose fluid, so don't drink to replace every ounce lost. (The glycogen and associated stored water that you expend over the course of a marathon can add up to four pounds.) We are designed to do this safely as long as we replace fluids later, at a meal, for instance. (That's what the post-race party is for.)
- Manage your electrolytes (critical during events of four to five hours, especially), as this will help maintain better fluid balance. During a race, you can drink small amounts of sports beverages to get some electrolytes. Better yet are electrolyte tablets, gels, or powdered mixes (I prefer UCAN Hydrate). Even the anticipation of food and water—swishing a carb drink, for instance—gives your brain a boost. (Rehearse this before the race.)
- Turn off your watch and let common sense set your pace. Anticipate at least a 2 percent drop in speed for every increment of 9°F (5°C) over an ambient temperature of 54°F (12°C).
- Dress white and light, and pretest how your shoes and socks perform when they are wet. (I don't wear socks, and run in light, minimalist shoes or sandals, so this isn't an issue for me.)
- Be smart. *Don't* run in the heat if you are poorly conditioned, have existing medical problems, use dietary supplements (especially stimulants), have a history of heat illness, or are taking prescription medications that affect heat regulation.

A few words on racing in the cold

The 2018 Boston Marathon provided an opportunity to experiment with the flip side of racing in the heat. Thirty thousand runners were served with pelting rain, a brutal 30 mph headwind, and a thermometer that never rose above 35°F. It was the perfect formula for super-cooling the body, short of jumping into the just-thawed Charles River. *The Boston Globe* counted 2,500 runners (including 25 elite racers) seeking treatment in the medical tent, mostly for hypothermia, and 5 percent of the starting runners, including many pre-race favorites, failed to complete the course. The fastest finish times came in 10 to 15 minutes slower than usual for Boston. Desiree Linden, the first American female winner in thirty-three years, came in at 2:39—a quarter hour off the average of recent years' winning times for women. The men's winner, Yuki Kawauchi, finished 10 minutes slower than the usual winner's time—while humbling the field by beating his closest challenger by 4 minutes. I ran it in 3:04, my slowest-ever marathon. But I was proud, if I may say so, that a dose of grit (and some race smarts and experience) kept me from the medical tent.

In hypothermia-inducing conditions, the most important strategy is to keep your core warm and dry. Here are a few simple tips:

- Trust the weather forecast, and get the right gear. Tech shirts alone will not repel the rain, so get a good running jacket (or at least a vest). In Boston I used an awesome jacket made by On.
- A good base layer is essential. The best I've found is made by XOSKIN, a U.S. company.
- Wear a hat, gloves, and even a hood (for the rain).
- Cut the wind on your face and exposed skin by applying sunscreen or olive oil. It keeps the cheeks warm and happy.
- Stay warm and dry before the start: wear plastic bags over your shoes, and anything to protect you from the cold, wind, and water. Trash liners can work (which you can recycle).
- Try consuming warm drinks and a few extra calories of food before the start. In cold weather your body burns extra fuel to simply maintain normal body temperature.

- Keep moving. Movement generates heat. If you stop, you'll start shivering.
- At the finish, quickly recover your warmth! I've found that a post-race hot shower (or even better, a sauna—a friend's hotel in Boston this year had one), will jump-start normal life again.

Below is my kit for the Boston Marathon 2018. It's not pretty, but it worked: XOSKIN base layer, On running jacket, hood, hat, gloves, sunscreen on face and legs, calf sleeves, and grit.

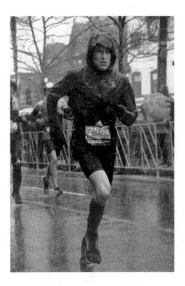

CHAPTER 13

The Runner's High:
The Mind of a Winner

Running has made being depressed impossible. If I'm going through something emotional and just go outside for a run, you can rest assured I'll come back with clarity.

—ALANIS MORISSETTE, singer and actress

Running is how I get a front-row seat to the calming, enjoyable spectacle of experiencing endorphins as they do their magical tap-dance inside my brain.

—BILL KATOVSKY, author,
co-founder of Natural Running Center

For every runner who tours the world running marathons, there are thousands who run to hear the leaves and listen to the rain, and look to the day when it suddenly is as easy as a bird in flight.

—GEORGE SHEEHAN, M.D.

MYTH: *Running is painful and exhausting.*

FACT: *Running can be fun and relaxing, and it enhances the production of brain-derived neurotrophic factor (BDNF), which stimulates cognitive ability, long-term memory, and the growth of new neurons.*

Those of us who run daily know what it's like to miss a day or two. A feeling of restlessness—for some, even pain or anxiety—sets in, growing into a compulsion to duck out of a meeting, to get moving, to stretch, to exert, to breathe, to be outside. Finally, once out and running, the cluttered mind clears. A feeling of calmness and relief flows in.

Despite the tendency to view running as painful and masochistic, the sheer abundance of dedicated runners (some of them even run through injury and illness) suggests that it *must* have a pleasurable and rejuvenating net effect. Whatever suffering we endure while running is almost always temporary, and when done right is virtually nonexistent. Yet the mental effects—relaxation, enhanced mood, and focus—linger long afterward.

Indeed, running can be addictive. Researcher David Raichlen and colleagues identified a variety of neurological rewards that are generated by running and by extended aerobic activity. The neurotransmitters dopamine, serotonin, norepinephrine, and acetylcholine are released, along with hormonal growth factors and endocannabinoids, which are related to the active compounds in marijuana. The exercise-activated surge of these chemicals plays a major role in stimulating the receptors in the pleasure centers of the brain. Together, these neurochemicals and their effects serve to boost our calming, *parasympathetic* tone.

HIT ME WITH SOME NEUROTRANSMITTERS

Sporadic exercise by people who are mostly sedentary isn't enough to release these neurochemicals. For some, walking isn't quite sufficient. There may be a threshold of time and intensity—a minimum time off the couch, in effect—that must be crossed before this marvelous physiological response kicks in. The tragedy here is that sedentary folks who find exercise uncomfortable (i.e., difficult to initiate or maintain) may be succumbing to inertia *just short of the threshold* at which the pleasure-inducing neurotransmitters start to flow. They are within arm's length of reaching the pot at the end of the rainbow. (Statin medications, especially in high-potency doses, may hold many back from reaching this threshold as well.)

THE RUNNER'S HIGH TIMES . . .

The term "runner's high" has stuck with us over the decades, but as running author Jim Fixx wrote in 1978 in the *New York Times,* "The effects of running are nothing like those resulting from use of alcohol or marijuana. While running, a person feels perfectly sober. Having showered and dressed, he or she can work as a doctor, stockbroker, teacher, lawyer, or whatever, with no adverse effects."

Fixx went on to write, "Where runners differ from other people, in addition to having efficient cardiovascular systems, is in the euphoric tranquility that is derived from the sport. What a runner feels is not unlike the serenity accrued from a few days' vacation. The difference is that the runners can summon this feeling whenever they want. Moreover, they do not have to fly to Aruba to find it."

Dogs share our addictive response to exercise—hence their frantic impatience, when kept indoors for long periods, to run and play outside. Like humans, dogs enjoy variety, which is why you don't see them electing to run around in circles or on a treadmill.

EXERCISE IS FOOD FOR THOUGHT

What are some of the other beneficial effects of aerobic physical activity?

Briefly, one is *angiogenesis,* or the growth of new blood vessels and capillaries. This improves blood flow, enhances oxygen and nutrient delivery, and improves the metabolic system's ability to "take out the garbage," or process toxic waste products.

Another benefit is *neurogenesis,* or the growth of new neurons in the brain. Exercise enhances neurotrophic growth factors, which are like brain fertilizer. In particular, BDNF, or brain-derived neurotrophic factor, boosts neurogenesis at the same time that it nourishes existing neurons, and is associated with cognitive improvement and the alleviation of depression and anxiety. Among those who exercise regularly, BDNF levels remain high even when at rest, and will stay high into advanced age as long as a routine of exercise is maintained. (It's likely that, as in mice, exercise increases the size and number of mitochondria in the hippocampus, where memories are formed and stored.)

No wonder that exercise improves memory and makes you feel better. Exercise may not make you smarter, but your cognitive abilities will improve. And if you fear dementia, don't stop running. You can even grow new brain cells in your eighties—with exercise. Healthy lifestyle choices (especially exercise) reduce your odds of developing dementia by up to 60 percent. (Note that there is a dose response to exercise: the benefits increase significantly for up to an hour or two of moderate activity a day. Added benefits taper off above that.)

The brain can adapt to a remarkable degree. The concept of neuroplasticity is now making its way into conventional treatments of dementia, Parkinson's, and stroke. Columbia University psychiatrist Norman Doidge describes what he terms "learned nonuse." An injury, disease, or stroke, for example, can shut off signaling to the part of the brain that controls movement of a specific area. But when we continually stimulate the interrupted motor circuits and patterns, the brain—because of its neuroplasticity—develops new circuits to work around the faulty ones.

Doidge emphasizes that aerobic exercise in particular promotes the health of two types of cells in the brain—neurons and glial cells (which protect the neurons)—while expanding the gray and white matter in the frontal lobes, which are regions that involve planning and goal-directed thinking.

IT TAKES GUTS TO ADAPT

Much of current medicine is based on a model of the body as a machine, and treatments are crafted in the manner of engineering diagrams. But we are biological beings, not mechanical models. We know that the impossibly complex human body is an organism with parts that can change, adapt, and grow. Indeed, not all of these parts are really "ours." The microbiome—the remarkable wealth of flora and fauna in our guts—is one of the new frontiers of research, and we're learning how it affects our metabolism, resistance to disease, and even our mood. (A greater quantity of serotonin, for instance, is produced in our internal biotic environment than is released by our nervous system.)

Can the organisms living in our guts actually affect the way we feel (and maybe even our body weight)? The gut is not simply an entryway for nutrients. Our intestines offer the largest surface area of interface between ourselves and the outside environment (more than the skin, for example). Trillions of organisms are harbored here, and they regulate and interact metabolically with our nervous and endocrine systems. The human microbiome has even been described as the "second brain" or "second endocrine system." The microbiology isn't well understood, but a healthy gut is an indicator of a healthy brain and good hormonal function. This emerging topic is explored in detail in the books and peer-reviewed articles of bacteriologist Dr. Martin Blaser and neurologist Dr. David Perlmutter.

ENGAGE STRESS TO DESTRESS

Everyone wants to avoid stress. In addition to the psychological hazards, chronic stress (a heightened state of cortisol production) leads to greater insulin resistance and enhanced production of betatrophin, a protein that blocks an enzyme that metabolizes body fat. This reduces metabolic efficiency, while making it harder to lose weight.

But is all stress bad?

A moderate exposure to stress is needed to survive and thrive. According to Dr. Kelly McGonigal (*The Upside of Stress: Why Stress Is Good for You, and How to Get Good at It*), it's the way we perceive stress and respond to it (and how long it lasts) that makes the difference.

If you think your stress is going to kill you, it just might. When stress is perceived as negative, with a feeling of loss of control, then the fight-or-flight (adrenaline) response is activated for prolonged periods. Cortisol, other glucocorticoids, and clotting factors are stimulated. Severe sympathetic stress can even switch off neurotrophic growth factors, to the degree that even exercise won't restore a stable state. You end up marinating your daily life in a damaging biochemical stew.

Dr. McGonigal offers some straightforward advice: view your body's stress response as vital to your health, as something that will make you stronger. Envision the stress as helping you to manage, learn from, and grow. Then you must relax. Your stressful, crazy life is not unique. Moderate stress should be welcomed as a daily challenge—as long as it doesn't control you.

When lions spot their prey, they're not thinking about resting. And when they are resting, they're not thinking about their next prey. Humans, on the other hand, seem to have it backward: when we're resting, we think inordinately about our stress, and when we are stressed we become fixated on resting.

EXERCISE FOR ANXIETY AND DEPRESSION

When you suffer physical or mental stress (which can be caused by *in*activity), you may seek relief through medications. But when we look carefully at a broad range of studies on the effectiveness of pharmacotherapy for stress, depression, anxiety, and cognitive impairment, drugs offer little, if any, benefit. (Pharmaceutical companies often design their own trials, and they publish and promote results selectively. Studies with negative or questionable results often go unpublished.)

The use of drugs can lead to dependence, side effects, downregulation of response (the drugs become less effective), and relapse. At best, they simply aren't as effective as physical activity (and healthy eating, and sleep) at expanding the beneficial neurotransmitter delivery system. When consistent exercise is part of a treatment plan for these disorders, relapse is uncommon—especially in comparison to medications and most other conventional therapies. Among committed runners and athletes, mood disorders are rare. A crowdsourced hub for patients' perspectives on effective (and ineffective) treatments can be found at a site called CureTogether.

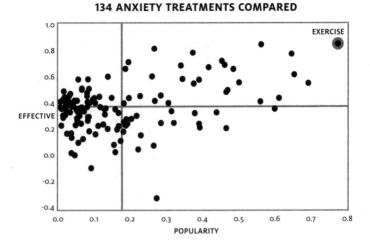

134 ANXIETY TREATMENTS COMPARED

This chart is based on nearly 32,000 people who self-reported suffering from anxiety. In the aggregate, exercise was the clear winner in terms of both effectiveness and popularity.

RUNNING FROM ADDICTION, ADDICTED TO RUNNING

In West Virginia, as around the nation, opiate addiction, mostly from opioid-based prescription drugs, has destroyed lives and families. What's supremely frustrating is that it is difficult to treat. I'm sometimes asked if I know anyone who has been weaned successfully from opiates without substitution of another drug (which is usually opioid-based, too).

I know of one person. Travis Muehleisen hadn't chosen to take pain meds. In 1997 and 2004, physicians prescribed them following back surgeries from spinal stenosis, which he acquired from injuries while working in the steel industry. After being disabled in 2007, he had two more back surgeries and was prescribed more drugs. Over that period, he became severely depressed, grew obese (330 pounds), and developed high blood pressure and coronary artery disease.

"I didn't care for this way of life," he told me, "but I knew no other way." After thirteen years of opiate addiction and declining health, he knew that he had to change or he would die.

Travis is now addicted to running. "In 2010, I began walking on the treadmill in my sister's basement, a mile at a time. Within a month, I worked up to three miles. Then I began running around the local high school track, a lap at a time. One month later, I ran four laps—a mile. Gradually I increased my distance, and in 2011 I ran my first half marathon."

He combined exercise with healthful eating and lost more than a hundred pounds. He no longer takes medications, and has returned to working full time. In an 8K race, he placed within the top 10 percent of his age group, then followed that with a marathon—26.2 miles—which he finished without stopping. In the past four years he has run sixteen marathons, and in 2017 he ran the JFK 50 Mile—only to miss the time cut, at the 46-mile mark, by a minute.

For Travis, running means going all in. If he doesn't run, and run hard, he literally feels pain. It takes a run of six miles, he told me, before sufficient endorphins kick in to act as an opiate substitute for him. *Endorphin* means "endogenously produced morphine." *You* produce the morphine.

Travis is the only person I know to work his way off disability (despite the disincentive to work when getting a paycheck not to). Desk job? No way. Travis builds bridges. He needs to work to keep his brain and body engaged. He's been free of opiates for seven years.

I asked him what he had learned over the past two decades. "Running has shown me that you can be stable and productive after addiction. If you want a good life bad enough, it's up to you to take control of it. You have to believe in yourself, recover your self-esteem, and mend the damage you have caused to family and friends. Find something that challenges you physically and mentally, and dive in."

FUSION ENERGY

Indeed, the biggest benefit of running may come down to self-confidence and peace of mind. In 1978, Dr. George Sheehan—a cardiologist-runner who became a writer after tiring of continually referring patients for bypass surgery—daringly suggested that most runners don't really run in order to become healthy. In examining their motivations, he classified runners into three groups: (1) A *jogger* is someone who is "born again" physically, and seeks to convert and reform by preaching running's benefits of longevity and reduced heart disease. As new challenges arise, the jogger desires to be (2) a *competitor,* which offers him an even longer break from the office or a boring daily routine. This stage chooses performance over health, and no sacrifice is too great. Then the jogger or competitor who is no longer obsessed with specific health benefits, and no longer needs the excitement of events, becomes (3) a *runner.* Finally, she sees running in perspective, Sheehan explains, as "the fusion of body, mind and soul in beautiful relaxation."

REBOOTING IS NOT JUST CHANGING YOUR FOOTWEAR

Most of us wouldn't benefit from trying to follow the stress-inducing regimen and schedule of an elite athlete. I maintain a fairly high level of fitness and run competitively, but I regard running (I deliberately shun the word "training") mainly as my daily *reset button.*

The harder and busier the day, the more I look forward to a run, and the more relaxation and immunity from stress I derive from it. Running is the perfect response to being overextended in work and life. (If running somehow brought on *more* stress, it simply wouldn't be sustainable.) Nowadays, busy, challenging lives are the norm. Running must fit seamlessly—and voluntarily—into the weekly schedule. Most important, it must make us feel better.

DRILLS

Breathe
One of the best stress-reduction exercises—which can be done at work and throughout the day—is relaxed abdominal breathing. Breathe in through your nose and fill your belly completely, then exhale fully with pursed lips, as if inflating a balloon. Work up to five seconds for each inhale, hold it for a few seconds, then ten seconds for the exhale. Notice your pulse drop as your parasympathetic system kicks in.

Run for stress relief
More than 85 percent of runners run to relieve stress. One simple drill is to *focus purely on releasing stress* while you run. Find a quiet, calming route. Focus on relaxed, rhythmic breathing. If you like running in a group, meet up and join them. I have a small group of busy friends, and every week or two we meet up for an early-morning run in a natural setting.

Be a lion
A few times a week, do something with high intensity, even if brief. My favorites are sprints and burpees. Knock off a few of these, just enough for a bit of fatigue. It invariably has a calming and rejuvenating effect.

Zone out
Running can be a great escape, a chance to "zone out." Plug into some music, a podcast, or an audiobook, and distract yourself from worries, obligations, endless to-do lists, and the monotony that can accompany a long run.

Zone in
Be 100 percent present, and deeply connect to the moment. Running makes an ideal movement meditation, beautiful in its simplicity and accessibility. Practice mindfulness by simply observing. (This may be especially relevant when you are trail running.) Embrace whatever appears before you and whatever sensations, thoughts, and emotions arise.

(*Zoning out* and *zoning in:* With thanks to Elinor Fish, author of *The Healthy Runner's Manifesto*. As Elinor says, "Stop striving and start thriving.")

Sleep

Sleep builds our capacity to respond and adapt quickly to a stress. There's no substitute. Relax, and do it well and completely.

CHAPTER 14

Outsmart Injuries with Prevention

Why are pain and movement linked? In the presence of acute injury and/or pain, if the nervous system concludes there is a threat to the tissues, then movement is the primary mechanism by which the nervous system can react to that threat.
—*Grieve's Modern Musculoskeletal Physiotherapy*

MYTH: *Running wears out the joints.*

FACT: *Joints benefit greatly from stress and impact, in the right amounts.*

More than half of all runners are injured each year.

Let's take a look at one subset of active people: enlisted men and women in our Air Force. In 2010, running ranked only behind basketball as the leading source of injuries. (Many of those b-ball injuries are running-related, too.) But that's minor compared to what the armed services see overall. The Department of Defense reported 8.3 million days of missed duty between 2005 and 2009 from *preventable musculoskeletal injuries.* These include overuse injuries, sprains, strains, dislocations, tears (ACL/cartilage), and spine problems, costing the military $1.5 billion a year in labor replacement, medical care, and long-term disability.

CHASED BY AMBULANCES

What's going on with all this injury? Why do so few medical studies adequately explain their complicated causes, and why does the medical profession offer little beyond reactive, symptomatic treatment? Running injuries are typically treated with rest, ice, injections, painkillers, stretching, MRIs, fancy tests, and various devices and shoe orthotics. But despite all this medical "care," evidence-based trials show that much of it doesn't work. Runners continue to get injured at consistently high rates.

I find this heartbreaking. It's too easy a progression for an injured runner to become a *former* runner. When we are offered only drugs, cumbersome interventions, and ineffective treatment for pain or injury, quitting running is a logical response.

SHIFTING THE KINETIC CHAIN OF COMMAND

Runners are at fault, too, though not intentionally. When we feel pain or an incipient injury, we tend to shift our gait or posture. But a compensation like this (along with the drugs or orthotics) can hide the original condition or trigger another injury in a different area of the body. Sometimes a domino effect of injury works its way up (or down) the body's kinetic chain.

Injuries seldom happen in isolation, and never without cause. I often see runners suffering from a cascade of injuries; finding the root cause requires tracing back through the series of accommodations the runner has made. Not uncommonly, a debilitating injury starts with something seemingly benign, such as a single ill-fitting shoe. Over time, this can progress to weakness and lack of control of the foot, which can cause or contribute to lower back pain.

As I work with a runner, I try to determine which tissues feel pain, and when and where onset of pain occurs. Some areas are more sensitive than others, such as the fascia of the feet, the small tendon insertions, and the lumbar fascia of the back. Pain in the joints and bones tends to appear later, as a delayed response, and it's not unusual to develop knee or hip arthritis, for instance, before the area becomes painful. In the case of stress fractures (especially in the foot), pain might arise only after the injury has progressed—and sometimes when bone scans or MRIs show multiple asymptomatic (painless) stress on the *opposite* side, distant from the affected, painful area. In other words, runners can injure themselves without feeling pain. Unaware of a developing injury, they run themselves into a fully injured state.

Too often, the sports medicine industry is inadvertently (or intentionally) complicit in all this pain and injury. Sports medicine responds efficiently to dramatic, gladiator-style trauma and orthopedic injuries. For a blown-out knee from a football tackle, for example, repair teams can rebuild you. But for injuries suffered from thousands of slightly misaligned micromovements, or repetitive stress, we are way behind. And, as we saw in chapter 11, standard treatments such as ibuprofen, naproxen, and other NSAIDs actually *inhibit* healing.

All of this underscores how essential it is for us to maintain—*on our own, without too much intervention*—the delicate relationship between our interconnected moving parts. It's mainly up to each of us to build the ability to respond to and prevent injuries. Running should not cause injury. It should make us injury-resistant, and injury-resilient. We run so we *don't* get hurt.

AVOID THE LOADING ZONE

Fortunately, progressive-minded physical therapists and biomechanists have begun to teach running technique as part of their treatment for injured runners. In one study, Irene Davis, director of the Spaulding National Running Center, had subjects run in minimal shoes and bare feet on a specially configured treadmill that could measure ground impact forces. The runners were told to land softly and quietly, to increase their step count, and to listen to their own real-time feedback on landing patterns. She found that these subtle adjustments helped them to significantly lower impact forces on their lower legs, reduce pain, and (in some cases) resolve chronic injuries. This technique for modifying gait is called *impact moderating behavior* (IMB)—an important term that I hope will gain currency among everyone who runs.

Elite athletes mostly know this. Those who don't have short careers. The wise ones learn that whenever they sense pain or discomfort, they need to understand the cause, address it, and encode IMB into their landings—not treat it symptomatically or surgically or rely on a shoe or insert to correct it.

I learned this the hard way myself. Earlier in my running years, I suffered a condition called hallux rigidus, in which I couldn't dorsiflex (bend upward) either big toe—a result of degenerative changes likely caused by running too hard, with poor form, in overdesigned and poorly fitting shoes. Surgery relieved some of the pain, and some mobility returned, but the joint remained mostly fused. Doctors suggested that I quit running.

CHANGE MUST COME FROM WITHIN

Inexplicably, after surgery on my feet, no one prescribed foot strengthening exercises or physical therapy, which is the treatment for other sports injuries. I knew that I needed exercise, and I found nothing as convenient or relaxing as running. (My dog missed it, too.) So rather than quit running, I set out to retool the way I ran.

At the time, I lived in Denver near a wooded park that featured a 2.5-mile running loop with a forgiving crushed rock surface. Initially, I harbored only one objective: to get out and enjoy myself. I now believe this to be the most meaningful and sustainable goal that any runner can have.

Running at slow speeds gave me the space to breathe, and the time to explore commonsense techniques of impact moderating behavior. I tried shorter strides (with a quicker cadence), and landed with knees bent and feet closer to my center of mass. I began to understand what *not* to do, such as land hard on my heels. I experimented with running methods. *ChiRunning* helped me learn new things: it stressed biomechanics, not workouts, and taught me to approach running as a complete practice, not as a sequence of disconnected movements.

PREHAB, NOT REHAB

Running injuries aren't inevitable. Most injuries are a product of *too much, too soon, too hard,* or *too fast.* Or a combination of these. We can prevent injuries in the first place by doing *prehab:* realigning the body's symmetry, maintaining posture, strengthening the feet, expanding the range of movement, learning gentle rhythm and relaxation, and remodeling movement patterns. *Treat the posi-*

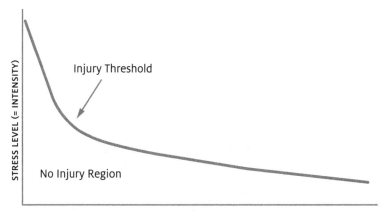

STRESS LEVEL (= INTENSITY)

Injury Threshold

No Injury Region

WORKOUT FREQUENCY

A low volume of high-intensity exertion can move someone above
the injury threshold. Likewise, so can large doses of low-intensity work.
The goal is to gradually elevate the injury threshold, with workouts
of low to medium intensity and duration.

tion, not the condition. The time to fix the roof, as JFK said, is when
the sun is shining.

We can also deter injury by unbinding and loosening physical restrictions, and building mobility—through careful mobility work and foam rolling. (Too much *stretching*, however, can be
counterproductive. Picture trying to undo the knot of a rope by
pulling it tighter.)

Your level of exertion affects vulnerability to injury, too. When
you're not overexerting (i.e., when you're running within the comfortable, aerobic zone), you can better feel discomfort and sense
incorrect form, and better judge when to stop. High-intensity running, by contrast, allows the hormones produced during the sympathetic, fight-or-flight response to mask structural pain. If you are
running above your maximum aerobic heart rate, you may wake
up surprisingly sore the next morning, or even find that you have
an injury.

The prescription for healthy running, when starting from an
injury-free state, is reasonably easy to fill: as you begin an exercise
routine, progress gradually. Walking injuries are rare, so don't be
afraid to start by walking. Then progress to a walk/jog mix, and
graduate to running.

WHAT ARE THE MOST COMMON
RUNNING INJURIES WE SEE?

There isn't room here to discuss every running injury. Our attention, anyway, should remain on turning off the faucet, not on mopping up the mess. Medical counsel can appear contradictory: on the one hand, most injuries are curable without medical intervention. But on the other, if you are severely injured and in pain you should seek help from a medical professional who understands running.

Let's take a look at the typical running injuries physicians see, and what can be done to treat them "post-actively" (for those of us who fell behind the prevention curve and exceeded the injury threshold). If you highlight a map of the body with common running injury hot spots (page 219), you'll see that the feet, lower legs, knees, and back light up most vividly.

Problem knees account for a large percentage of running injuries every year. Common knee and upper leg conditions include:

- *Iliotibial band syndrome (ITBS)*—pain on the lateral (outside) aspect of the knee.
- *Patellofemoral pain syndrome (PFPS)*—pain on the underside of the patella.
- *Hamstring sprains/strains*—injury is usually where the hamstring crosses joints (knee and hip); most injuries occur high in the hamstring.

Foot, ankle, and lower leg problems account for another large percentage of running injuries. The four most common of these conditions are:

- *Achilles tendinosis*—chronic inflammation and degeneration of the Achilles tendon.
- *Plantar fasciosis*—degeneration and microtears of the plantar fascia of the foot.
- *Medial-tibial stress syndrome* (commonly referred to as shin splints)—usually early stage microfractures that occur along the inside edge of the tibia.

RUNNING INJURIES
Causes and Symptoms

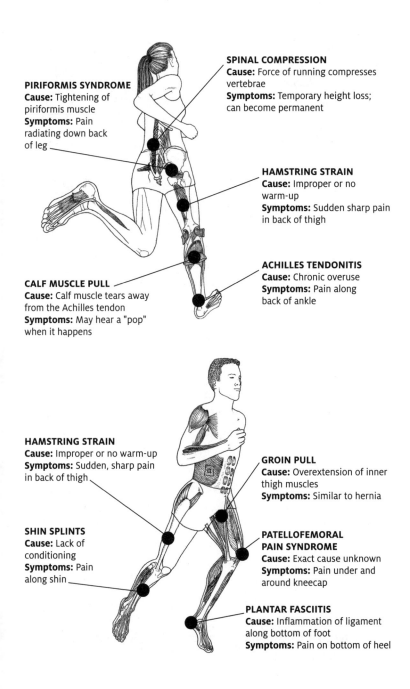

PIRIFORMIS SYNDROME
Cause: Tightening of piriformis muscle
Symptoms: Pain radiating down back of leg

SPINAL COMPRESSION
Cause: Force of running compresses vertebrae
Symptoms: Temporary height loss; can become permanent

HAMSTRING STRAIN
Cause: Improper or no warm-up
Symptoms: Sudden sharp pain in back of thigh

CALF MUSCLE PULL
Cause: Calf muscle tears away from the Achilles tendon
Symptoms: May hear a "pop" when it happens

ACHILLES TENDONITIS
Cause: Chronic overuse
Symptoms: Pain along back of ankle

HAMSTRING STRAIN
Cause: Improper or no warm-up
Symptoms: Sudden, sharp pain in back of thigh

GROIN PULL
Cause: Overextension of inner thigh muscles
Symptoms: Similar to hernia

SHIN SPLINTS
Cause: Lack of conditioning
Symptoms: Pain along shin

PATELLOFEMORAL PAIN SYNDROME
Cause: Exact cause unknown
Symptoms: Pain under and around kneecap

PLANTAR FASCIITIS
Cause: Inflammation of ligament along bottom of foot
Symptoms: Pain on bottom of heel

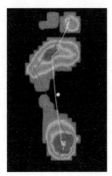

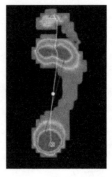

Assessing the foundation: at Two Rivers Treads we use a plantar pressure map to assess and retrain the foot to proper shape, strength, and balance.

- *Stress fractures*—progressed microfractures that most commonly occur in the tibia, metatarsals, or calcaneus.

Generally, muscle injuries occur when one's range of motion is exceeded, and when tissues are abnormally stressed. Bone and joint injuries tend to result from high or repetitive impact (abnormal loading).

Knee valgus is the motive force behind the epidemic of non-contact anterior cruciate ligament (ACL) injuries in jumping and explosive sports such as basketball, volleyball, and skiing. Less commonly, ACL injuries can also occur from lower-impact, high-repetition movements, such as running.

The relatively new regimen of core and hip training is designed to deal with valgus movement, by stabilizing the stance and preventing the femur from rotating inward on landing. Despite a decade of experience in the athletic community with this core and hip training, however, valgus-related injury rates are still high. Curiously, in the early days of running, these injuries were rare—most people simply ran correctly. Little attention was given to accessory core training, and if runners wanted to build strength, they ran and bounded up hills.

Dynamic knee valgus, it turns out, typically begins with the foot. The knee is more like the kid caught in the middle: it's only doing what the hip and the foot tell it to. A weak and unstable foot—one that can't control impact loads, then collapses—takes the knee along with it.

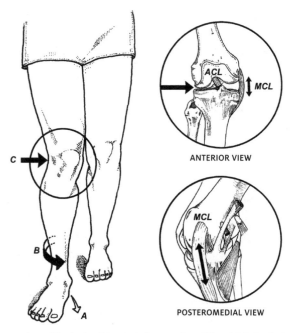

The image above illustrates "dynamic knee valgus," in which the knee dives inward in an "L" shape, commonly seen during high-impact movements such as jumping and landing. Movement sequence A → B → C can lead to anterior cruciate ligament (ACL) and medial collateral ligament (MCL) tears.

If the hip is strong and the foot is weak, the knee will collapse. This is one reason why I don't recommend shoes with excessive support or marshmallow-soft cushioning. The foot is your foundation, and it needs to be strong and solidly planted on the ground.

PLANTAR FASCIOSIS—A LIFESTYLE INJURY

Plantar fasciosis is not primarily a running injury—it's a common malady. But every week or so, the Natural Running Center receives a query from a reader desperate for relief from chronic plantar fasciosis pain. Fortunately, the approach to treating it is fairly straightforward, and can be applied to other injuries. (Technically, *fasciosis* refers to a degeneration of the tissue, which is far more common than *fasciitis*—the conventionally used term. Fasciitis implies true inflammation, and occurs in situations such as infection or auto-immune attack. Similarly, Achilles *tendonosis* is more common than *tendonitis*.)

The strong, springy plantar fascia tendon maintains the arch of the foot. It creates tension between the calcaneus (heel) and the metatarsal heads, forming the depressable arch that acts as the foot's primary spring, like a leaf spring on a car.

The plantar fascia is designed to manage a limited amount of stress. The intrinsic muscles (those solely in the foot) and extrinsic muscles (those attaching the foot to the lower leg) receive signals from the nerves and fascia, and it's these muscles that should absorb and manage most of the load. When those muscles become dysfunctional or weak, the load is transferred to the plantar fascia, where repetitive stress causes microtrauma, and eventually plantar fasciosis.

Plantar fasciosis tends to recur, for the simple reason that sports medicine does little to prevent it. I suffered from it for years, such that even walking became a miserable, painful experience. Injections, night splints, over-the-counter arches, rigid custom arches, stable shoes, stretching—nothing helped. If shock wave therapy had been in vogue, I'm sure I would have tried it.

For sufferers like me, typical first treatments include arch supports or NSAIDs, neither of which are effective in the long term. Arch supports may provide some relief, but they only serve to *brace and weaken* the arch. (Some structural foot deformities can benefit from supports.) Always, the goal is improvement in function and strength. Anti-inflammatories only circumvent the natural repair process, and pain recurs as soon as the stress is reapplied.

The only way to sustainably fix plantar fasciosis is to address the root causes. Is the runner suffering from *fallen* arches, or is it *failing* arches? Gradually reducing and removing arch supports, while building foot strength and moderating impact, is the best place to begin. Paradoxically, shoes that offer lots of support *weaken* the foot, causing more foot instability.

Other factors can contribute to plantar fasciosis, such as a misaligned and weak big toe, tight and shortened calf muscles, obesity, or transitioning too quickly from supportive footwear to flat shoes or bare feet.

Treatment for plantar fasciosis varies, depending on the cause, but as a general guideline:

- Orthotics such as arch supports or taping should be used only as a *temporary* modality while you strengthen and lengthen tissues. (You don't leave a broken arm in a cast forever; muscles begin to atrophy from disuse within a week.) Don't wear heels, and find shoes with wide toe boxes.
- Place your forefeet on a stair, and lower your heels, then raise them. It's fine to feel a bit of discomfort while doing this, as long as you are progressively increasing strength and control of the feet. This is great for the Achilles tendon, and the tibialis posterior muscle and tendon, too.
- Do some soft tissue work to loosen the plantar fascia if it is thickened, tight, and tender. Forcibly work the soles of your feet with your thumbs, rollers, or even golf balls, to release the fascia knots. Healthy fascia slides and glides.
- Work the intrinsic muscles of the feet. Pick things up with your feet. Walk barefoot. As often as you can, strengthen the muscles of the big toes by dorsiflexing them, then pressing them into the ground—toe yoga. This will awaken the foot muscles and help re-create the arch. The short foot posture exercises can be done throughout the day, too, even inside your (flexible) shoes. (Barefoot Science insoles can stimulate these muscles all day.)
- If your big toes are misaligned and bent inward (hallux valgus), which is common, consider using a product to straighten them, such as Correct Toes.
- Practice slow jogging, with lighter ground contact and loading rates. Relearn how to land and spring. Easy jump-roping teaches this, too.
- Avoid NSAIDs (naproxen, ibuprofen, etc.). These drugs interfere with natural healing processes, and can cause medical complications. In college, I suffered a bleeding ulcer from these meds, and lost over half my blood volume.

- Consult a health care provider who understands natural running and walking.

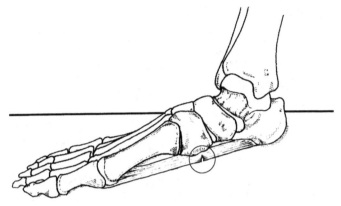

A collapsed foot creates strain and microtears of the plantar fascia.

HANDIATRY?

Why have our feet become such a problem, and why are there so many podiatrists? Look at your hands, and ponder why we don't have "handiatrists." It's because we utilize our hands daily for a wide variety of tasks. We run them through an extraordinary range of healthful motions—unencumbered by heavy, confining, posture-altering gear of the sort that we routinely wear on our feet. Remove the shoes or wear minimal ones, and many foot problems will go away (with time and patience).

RESET, NOT REST

Misperceptions abound. Some injuries require rest and rehabilitation, but many don't.

One runner, Natalee Maxfield, played on sports teams in high school, then picked up running in college, married, and ran throughout her pregnancies. In her thirties, she developed foot pain, which podiatrists variously ascribed to Morton's neuroma, plantar plate injury, and capsulitis. They prescribed rest and orthotics. But she didn't want to stop running.

Natalee sensed that she would need to find lasting relief on her own, and that the best therapy would be to simply not get injured in the first place. She adjusted her running style, switched to shoes with a more minimal profile, and hasn't been injured since. As Natalee and others have learned on their own, many running injuries require correct *remodeling,* not medical intervention or rest.

Any time a tissue endures strain (in which it is stretched and lengthened), it is deformed. Picture what happens when you bend a ski pole: under stress, it flexes and springs back to its original shape—up to a point. When *strained* or *over*stressed, it becomes stuck in a new, bent position, requiring that it be forcibly restraightened in order to be useful. This is what happens when a shoulder, for instance, is secured in a sling. In as little as three days it freezes in that position. The process of remodeling it correctly—getting it to work again through its full range of motion—is painful and difficult.

If you are suffering from a running-related pain, the joints—indeed, all parts of the body—generally benefit from *movement* of the affected area, *not immobilization.* Running (and walking) the *right* way is an excellent treatment for degenerative injuries sustained from running the *wrong* way. In my practice, I continually witness the body's remarkable ability to heal itself and restore itself to its natural position—while people remain active—if the causative issues are addressed and the right signals are sent.

Mistakenly, many of us are "rehabbing" basic movements and skills out of ourselves by focusing on an isolated exercise. Imagine seeking guidance from six golf swing coaches—a backswing coach, a stance coach, a strategist, and so on. You might succeed in improving the movement of a single specific muscle group, yet you'd still have a dysfunctional swing.

AS YOGI BERRA MIGHT HAVE SAID, HALF THE PAIN WE FEEL IS 90 PERCENT MENTAL

Pain management is a persistent challenge in the treatment of running injuries. And one of pain's enduring mysteries is the manner in which we *anticipate* it. (Note that it's the brain and nervous system that register and process pain, not the injured part.) Experiments have looked at how people respond to a painful stimulus applied to someone else's limb, or to a sham limb, that is placed in a position where it appears to be one's own. (See Dr. Lorimer Moseley's TED talk, "Why Things Hurt," linked on the videos page of runforyoulifebook.com.) PET scans show that subjects can experience genuine, objectively measurable pain—from a physical stimulus that doesn't exist.

Why do we feel pain in the first place? For one thing, it's a signal telling us that we need to protect tissue that is harmed or at risk. To the extent that it correctly alerts us to the problem, pain can protect us from further damage. But the signal can have a lag time, or come from an area that isn't the actual source of stress.

In other words, the patient and the doctor can misinterpret the signaled pain. Even worse, when doctors offer symptomatic treatment (the easy, billable solution), they leave the root cause of the pain unattended and untreated. The simple binomial that *pain is bad* and *relieving pain is good* is a simplistic response that seldom translates into appropriate medical treatment. Indeed, this approach has guided us directly into the current opioid addiction crisis.

When it comes to running, changing your mental approach can do wonders. Running coach Elinor Fish urges that simply shifting your mind-set from *running causes injury and pain* to *running makes me injury-resistant* will reduce your chances of developing an overuse injury. "With a positive mind-set," Elinor says, "you set the stage for establishing new habits that support running as a lifelong practice. While it's easy to view running as the cause of your injury, it's more likely that running is just making you aware of a preexisting problem. For example, sitting all day long causes chronic shortened hip flexors and underdeveloped glutes, both of which make running more difficult." The pain and stiffness and sensitivity arise when you are out running, so we don't automatically make the connection to the real cause: *sitting*.

AN EXPERIMENT OF ONE

Ultimately, a doctor or physical therapist can't know you intimately, and you need to rely on yourself as diagnostician and medical researcher—with yourself as the patient and experimental subject. Each of us responds differently to exercise, to physical stress, to the numerous insults that our bodies face as we move across the surface of the earth and interact with the objects on it. Ultimately, your personal experiment should seek one important outcome: to avoid injury. Do not put pain into your body. In place of the aphorism *No pain, no gain,* we should approach our activity with the conviction *No pain, thank you.*

DRILLS

Evaluating someone standing in a rested state provides a physical therapist with only part of a picture. The therapist—you, in this case, examining yourself—needs to see what happens under load, and especially in a fatigued state. Take a look at a sequence of pictures of yourself in a race: you look pretty good in the early images. By the end it's a different story. As you fatigue, your posture and form change—almost never for the better.

A high-speed smartphone camera can reveal a lot. Try video recording the following:

1. A single-leg step down from a low platform. Watch what is happening at the foot, the knee, and the hip. If the knee collapses inward, try to notice what gives out first. Is it the foot or the hip?
2. Ten hops on a single leg. This shows what happens under a bit of load. Then magnify the response and fatigue yourself by doing three or four minutes of shuttle runs, a few burpees, some jumps, and a few sprints. Then do the single-leg step down and single-leg hop tests again. Notice the difference? Even elite athletes will show weaknesses. (Do this fatigue test cautiously, and only if not injured.)

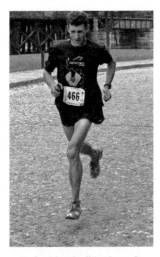

My foot lands directly under my hip, as if stomping grapes.

Identify and correct any "pathokinematic" (dysfunctional) movement pattern before you train for your next marathon. Build strength and follow gait cues. Don't overstride. From the frontal view, land with each foot directly under the hip (as if ascending stairs). Think of running on a line, with each foot landing on either side of the line, never touching it.

Inure yourself to injuries

The objective of the following drills is to protect yourself from injury and pain. Here are some simple ways to short-circuit the repetitive stress and high impact that typically result in injuries.

- Rather than run the same route each time you go out, alter the path you take. Changing up your route lets your body adapt to different environments. Trail running, for instance, improves balance and muscle strength (though it comes with the risks of unpredictable terrain). Soft grass or sand offers a cushioned landing for runners, but requires more muscle use, because there is less energy returned when your foot strikes the ground. Mix it up. Throw in some new challenges, and enjoy—but make the changes gradually.
- Transition—again, gradually—from a heavily cushioned and supportive shoe with an elevated heel to a minimal shoe that is flatter, lighter, thinner, wider, and more flexible. Your freed-up feet will thank you.
- Listen to your body. Don't mask discomfort with pain medication or anti-inflammatories. Slow down, add gentle and progressive stress, and recover. Then notice what you're no longer noticing: pain, soreness, and stiffness.
- Along with the TrueForm Runner (a remarkably useful tool for gait retraining and injury prevention), try the Zero Runner. This no-impact trainer allows for full range of motion in the hips, and *variability* of movement. (An elliptical trainer or Stairmaster, by contrast, dictates your movement.) If you are recovering from a stress fracture, joint replacement, or other mechanical stress or overload-related injury, the Zero Runner (which is great fun) can get you back in the game.

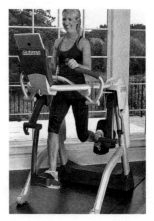

PART III

Running Is for Everyone

CHAPTER 15

Women Are Pulling Away from the Pack

If you want to become the best runner you can be, start now.
Don't spend the rest of your life wondering if you can do it.

—PRISCILLA WELCH,
winner of the New York Marathon, at age forty-three

Leave your watch on the kitchen table and go—freely, like a
child.

—CLAIRE KOWALCHIK,
The Complete Book of Running for Women

MYTH: *Running is mainly for men.*

FACT: *Today there are more women runners than men runners.*

MYTH: *Women shouldn't run when they are pregnant.*

FACT: *Women have run safely during pregnancy for as long as*
humans have been on the earth.

MYTH: *Women should not run if they have osteoporosis.*

FACT: *For osteoporosis, consistent, gradual exercise helps build*
bone strength and the balance that is needed to prevent falling.

This book is intended for everyone—men, women, and kids;
young and old. But there are some issues outlined in this chapter
that are specific to women.

One of the wildest tales of fiction, resulting in decades of lost opportunity for women in running, was the media coverage of the women's 800-meter race in the 1928 Olympics. "Below us on the cinder path were 11 wretched women," wrote John Tunis of the *New York Evening Post,* "5 of whom dropped out before the finish, while 5 collapsed after reaching the tape." His and other accounts described a "terrible exhaustion," which was widely accepted as an accurate depiction. As a result, the 800-meter distance for women was dropped from the Olympics until 1960.

The true story of 1928 is quite different, as shown in the film coverage linked on the book website's videos page. In those pretelevision and -Internet days, this footage would have been scarcely viewed. As is evident, only nine runners ran the race, and only one fell at the finish, then arose quickly. In this single event, several of them broke the existing women's 800-meter world record. They ran with grace and relaxation, and there were plenty of smiles at the finish.

For women, the 1,500-meter distance (just short of a mile) was included in the Olympics only in 1972, and the first women's marathon was run in 1984. The 10,000-meter race was added in 1988, the 5,000 meters in 1996, and the 3,000-meter steeplechase in 2008.

In 1966, female runner Bobbi Gibb petitioned to become an official entrant in the Boston Marathon. Race director Will Cloney responded with, "This is an AAU Men's Division race only . . . Women aren't allowed, and furthermore are not physiologically able."

Bobbi Gibb ran anyway.

The larger women's running movement, and the many changes made to racing rules, were driven primarily by brave women who simply desired to run, and to challenge themselves. Why obstruct anyone who seeks the pleasure, freedom, and health of running? By the 1980s, women posted times that would have beat or equaled the top male Olympians of a generation earlier.

This doesn't surprise me, especially after I had a chance, in 2001, to study the form of multiple world champion and Boston Marathon winner Catherine "the Great" Ndereba as I ran alongside her at the Boston Marathon. Until she pulled away, that is. I was with her group when we hit the halfway point in 1:14, and her light, springy stride and total relaxation seemed to propel her. In contrast, the body language and heavier breathing of those she left behind exposed their wasted energy. Catherine stayed relaxed on the long downhill, then tightened the screws and hugely accelerated over the Newton hills, running the final ten miles in 50 minutes, finishing in 2:24. Catherine helped my day. By cueing off her pacing and relaxation, I finished in 2:29—faster than I had expected, considering the surgery on my feet a year earlier.

IN IT TOGETHER

When friend and author Christopher McDougall came to Shepherdstown for a run and a talk over coffee, he described how 1992 Olympic gold medalist Derartu Tulu, of Ethiopia—at age thirty-seven, after childbirth and without having run a marathon in five years—returned to the endurance running circuit and ran the 2009 New York Marathon. From the start, she boldly took a position in the lead pack. As usual, the pack began dwindling as they entered Manhattan and ran up First Avenue. When they crossed over to the Bronx at Mile 20, the few who were able to stay with the lead pack appeared to struggle. That's when Derartu *slowed down and encouraged them to keep up*. After assisting and coaxing as much as she could, she pulled ahead and won the race.

South Africans often use the word *Ubuntu*, which translates as "I am because of you." In my experience, it is this quality that is central to the women's running movement.

TALKIN' 'BOUT THEIR GENERATION . . .

A new generation of women has become running's leading force, and more than 40 percent of marathon finishers are women. The half marathon is the fastest-growing competitive distance, and more than 60 percent of recent years' entrants are women—up from only 20 percent in 1985. Not only have their numbers increased, but their fastest times have improved at a faster rate than have men's times: the women's marathon record has dropped by *46 minutes* since the first sanctioned women's marathon, in 1972. Men's fastest marathon finishes have improved by less than 30 minutes over the past *century*.

In 1995, Oprah Winfrey entered, and handily completed, the Marine Corps Marathon. Pre-Oprah, races were for speedy folks. She proved that anyone—and women in particular—can go out and run. She characterized it correctly not as a sport but as a "healthy activity."

Of the millions of women who have taken up running, few have quit. Nudged along by the inevitable release of endorphins, most women run in a relaxed, contented style, less aggressively than men, with more consistent pacing. It's self-perpetuating: the act of running reinforces the desire to go out and do it again. For many mothers and other working women, running or exercising outdoors is the highlight of a busy day.

THE TORTOISES RELIABLY BEAT THE HARES

Men have a larger muscle mass—their testosterone advantage—meaning that they have a higher strength-to-weight ratio, and tend to be faster than women at short distances. But the performance gap between men and women diminishes in longer-distance events. A woman who equals a man at shorter distances will likely run as fast as, and often surpass, the same man when running longer distances. In ultra races, such as fifty miles and above, women in the 50th percentile of the women's results reliably outpace the men in their 50th percentile. Healthy women, with their higher natural percentage of body fat, can readily adapt to burn fat—the fuel that is needed for longer distances.

EAT (DIFFERENTLY) TO BE FIT

So, what are the specific medical issues that physically active women should be aware of?

A woman's hormonal changes through life (and a man's, to a lesser degree) include the upregulation of insulin resistance/carbohydrate intolerance. This means that many women can't get away with the same eating patterns when they enter their forties and fifties (and during pregnancy) as they did when they were younger and during preadolescence. Avoiding metabolic syndrome is of key importance as women age. It's not possible to outrun a bad diet.

Although obesity and diabetes are overwhelming health crises, and are likely to continue for some time, sports doctors see another, not uncommon condition in the form of what is called *relative energy deficiency in sport,* or RED-S (an emerging, broader term for what has long been called the *female athlete triad*).

This deficiency, or syndrome, is a cluster of symptoms and disorders that, when taken together, can result in poor health and adverse outcomes. It is seen most commonly among high-performing athletes, although symptoms and risk factors can be identified as early as middle school. RED-S tends to occur when three circumstances converge:

> *Nutritional imbalance or insufficiency.* This isn't necessarily an eating disorder. Gymnasts, ballet dancers—and long-distance runners—may sometimes appear unnaturally thin. Basically, they are struggling with an energy imbalance that develops when there is an energy or nutritional mismatch between the nutrients going in and what the sport and their bodies demand. For optimal bone and tissue growth, women require not only adequate calories but a well-balanced diet of essential fatty acids, essential amino acids, and the other nutrients that are obtained from real food.
> The body fat of a healthy female (with the capacity to have normal cycles and sustain a normal pregnancy) must be at least 20 percent of overall weight. Ballerinas, gymnasts, and elite runners often have body-fat levels well below this, sometimes dipping into the single digits. They are fit, but not always healthy. Our culture idealizes women who are ultra-thin, too, which likely contributes to the tendency toward nutritional imbalance.
> *Low bone density.* We lay down most of our bone matrix by the end of our teens. After that, bone cells (known as osteoclasts and osteoblasts) are broken down and rebuilt every day through a process of "remodeling," which is

acutely affected by the amount of impact loading. Impact and load-bearing sports, which help build and protect bone mineral density, are necessary and good—up to a point. Overloading causes more breakdown than buildup.

Low bone density, or osteopenia, can lead to increased risk of stress fractures, and is a precursor to osteoporosis. Osteopenia is seen more commonly among post-menopausal women as their estrogen levels naturally decline, and (of surprise to many) in swimmers, cyclists, and others engaging in non-weight-bearing activities.

Vitamin D (which is more of a hormone than a vitamin) also plays a role, as it is essential for building bone strength. Yet a study of women college athletes found that nearly a third of them were deficient in it. In addition, 30 percent of Division 1 female athletes were found to be iron deficient.

Menstrual dysregulation, or irregular ovulation. A regular menstrual cycle works as a regulator for normal metabolism and growth, and an environment of good nutrition and health is necessary to maintain this. With a regular cycle, the body produces the right hormones, in the correct amounts. When not regular, or in amenorrhea, the body is in a state of hormonal imbalance. Elite sports or dance performance, if requiring body fat below 20 percent, may be a mismatch for health.

Treating RED-S requires an adjustment to lifestyle that many find challenging. Once menstrual dysregulation has set in, it may take six to twelve months to restore healthy cycles, mainly by shifting gears from a state of physical overload and nutritional mismatch to a state of growth and repair. It's a matter of choosing health over fitness. For all the benefits of running for women's health, it's important to beware that too much running can cause problems, too.

To put it simply: eat healthfully and dial down the exercise. Bone remodeling and hormonal balance are keenly affected by the quality of one's nutrition, and improvement will occur from efforts in the kitchen. It's hard to get all the essential fats (especially omega-3s), amino acids, and B vitamins from a purely plant-based diet, so as a physician I don't encourage athletes (especially those engaging in high-impact activities) to go vegetarian or vegan. These diets can work in response to specific medical conditions (fasting can, too, in some cases), but we all need the full spectrum of building blocks, especially when active. If they do it scrupulously, athletes can train and compete on a vegetarian-only diet, but it is not the norm. Matt Fitzgerald (*The Endurance Diet*) traveled the globe to study the diets of the best athletes in all endurance sports. He did not find a single vegan athlete. Perhaps tellingly, traditional cultures reserve the richest, most nutrient-dense foods for women of childbearing age.

The stresses of life also stress your endocrine system. Find a trusted medical provider (an informed coach, trainer, sports nutritionist, or doctor) who can work with you through the recovery—especially someone who understands you and your commitment to sports.

THINGS CHANGE, ESPECIALLY IN ADOLESCENCE

For girls, the rapid changes that occur during adolescence don't always favor endurance or fast running speeds, and it's a time when many active young women ease away from sports. Fortunately, Title IX has helped to keep girls and women in the game.

The adolescent female gains body weight not from overeating but as a result of surges in the spectrum of hormones that drive growth, body shape change, and essential fat storage. Adolescent boys are growing and putting on weight, too, but their testosterone-dominant hormones direct more of this weight into muscle mass. (They don't grow because they are eating; they eat because they are growing.)

In other words, females' hormones prepare and reshape their bodies for childbirth, while males' surges of testosterone and growth hormone shape and prepare them for more physical tasks. A twin brother and sister may grow up sharing the same diet and activities, and enter adolescence with similar body forms and athletic skills. But they emerge from high school with completely different physical attributes and body fat percentages.

Peer pressure can be intense during adolescence, and young women are at risk for depression. This makes a simple activity such

Health consequences of relative energy deficiency in sport (RED-S) showing an expanded concept of the female athlete triad to acknowledge a wider range of outcomes and the application to male athletes.

(*Psychological consequences can either precede RED-S or be the result of RED-S.)

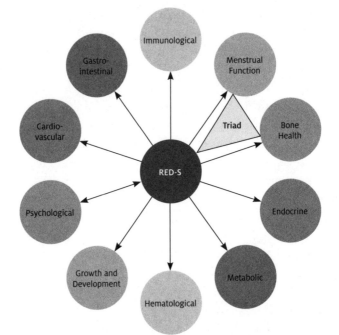

Relative energy deficiency in sport refers to impaired physiological function including (but not limited to) metabolic rate, menstrual function, bone health, immunity, protein synthesis, and cardiovascular health.

as running especially beneficial for overall health. During adolescence, physical activity is critical for the development of structural tissues such as bone, muscle, tendons, ligaments, and fascia. But it also enhances metabolism, brain function, mood, socialization, and quality of sleep. It even benefits the eyes, especially in this myopia-afflicted digital age. When you are running, your eyes strengthen by constantly changing focus between far, near, and peripheral distances—as contrasted with the rigidity of continual focus on a screen.

Different patterns of overuse injuries present in adolescent girls, too. As hips widen, foot and knee landing patterns can change, and knee valgus (the knee caving inward on landing) is all too common. "Runner's knee" (a general term that refers to pain in the knee), IT band syndrome, and other maladies around the knee travel with knee valgus, and are especially common among adolescent women.

CHANGING EXPECTATIONS WHEN EXPECTING

In traditional cultures, and until modern times, pregnancy was viewed as part of the cycle of a healthy woman's life. In many cultures still, women rarely change their activity levels in pregnancy. But when I began my medical career, restrictions during pregnancy (prescribed by white-coated "experts") began to creep in. Women were discouraged from running.

Few doctors noticed what is now becoming apparent: physically active women have better pregnancy outcomes. Fortunately, over the past couple of decades the experts have periodically relaxed earlier limitations on activity while pregnant. By 2018, we have finally agreed that it's best to simply use *good sense*. In other words, if running makes you happy and healthy, keep running. Run your first hundred-mile race while pregnant? Probably not good sense.

At the University of Colorado in the early 2000s, I worked in a wildly busy obstetrics fellowship for rural family physicians, delivering babies for mostly young Hispanic women. By and large, the mothers were healthy and enjoyed strong family support, and their labors and deliveries were mostly normal. Rarely did we need to intervene medically, and the C-section rate was in the single digits. In 2018, nearly a third of U.S. babies are now delivered by C-section.

THE OTHER CHANGE OF LIFE

Menopause presents its own challenges, in the form of depressed mood, fatigue, appetite changes, loss of desire, sleep disturbance, and a decline in youthful vitality. For decades, hormone replacement therapy (HRT) was routinely prescribed by doctors—until the Women's Health Initiative linked HRT to a slightly elevated risk for breast cancer and cardiovascular events. Ever since, the search has been on for safer alternatives such as antidepressants and nutritional and herbal remedies—with mixed results. If you're healthy, the increment of added risk from HRT may not be large, so evaluate your HRT options carefully with a trusted health care provider. Note that there's no evidence that HRT improves running performance.

Are there any risks of running during menopause, and later? Not in particular. You can expect mostly benefits, with no side effects or increased risks. But it's important to remain aware of RED-S and osteopenia, and work your way into a training program gradually. Distance running sensations Colleen De Reuck, Zola Budd, Joan Benoit Samuelson, and Meghan Arbogast continue to rewrite the understanding of what can be done after age fifty.

TAKIN' CARE O' BUSY-NESS

Running coach and author Elinor Fish has struggled with occasional fatigue, particularly as a parent. "As I get older and life seems to move ever faster, filled with more pressures and worries, fatigue issues arise more frequently. This can make it hard to run consistently, and at times has been so severe that it was all I could do to get through the workweek—in order to spend the entire weekend in bed. My poor husband had no idea how to help me.

"In response, I began to research stress. I was shocked to learn how profoundly stress affects the body and contributes to chronic health issues. I'm especially sensitive to this because I have an auto-immune condition that flares terribly when my stress levels rise."

Once Elinor started to actively manage her stress, she said, her vitality and desire to run began to return. Now many women runners who are facing the challenges of demanding jobs and family lives come to her with their stories of stress-induced and fatigue-related health problems. "Their busy schedules have left them with little time for self-care, including activities that relax the mind and restore their energy," Elinor said. "This is significant because women physically respond to stress differently than men do."

Elinor's experience aligns with that of Arianna Huffington, who in her book *Thrive* explains that women are paying a higher price than men for their participation in a workforce fueled by stress, sleep deprivation, and burnout.

THE MAGIC OF TWO FEET OFF THE GROUND

Is all of this running a good thing? Why do millions of women around the world take to running, and even endure injuries to keep doing it? Why not just walk, cycle, swim, train on an elliptical, or just squat repeatedly throughout the day?

My wife's cousin Meaghan Cusack exemplifies how our need for full mobility and body movement—of the kind that running provides—is ingrained in our DNA.

Meaghan describes her youth as not very athletic. "I dreaded the day in gym when we filed outside for the mile run. It was only four laps around the school, but it felt like a marathon." At the age of ten, she developed a pain in her ankle in gymnastics, and limped around for several weeks. Multiple ankle X-rays showed nothing. A few months later, she noticed a lump near her knee, and was diagnosed with osteosarcoma, an aggressive form of bone cancer.

More than two years of chemotherapy, relapses, and failed attempts at joint salvage finally came to a conclusion when doctors found that the cancer had spread to her lungs. It meant another year of chemotherapy.

Her leg had been valiantly trying to heal in the midst of it all, but the final year of chemo was the last straw. Her father was in tears when the doctor pulled up the X-ray of her lower leg. The bone was nearly gone, and they knew it would never heal. Two days later, the hospital room filled with family and friends who prayed over her as she was wheeled into surgery to amputate her leg above the knee.

Meaghan never allowed the disability to limit her goals. After graduating from college, she went on to get a master's and a Ph.D., while learning to walk on various prostheses and competing in cycling events. But she never *ran*. Until, that is, she met a prosthetist who asked her if she would ever want to try running again.

"I was hesitant at first," she said, "but he gave me a prosthetic running foot, and I took it home to try. Starting in the hallway of my building, I cautiously planted one foot in front of the other, then gradually lengthened my stride and increased my pace." Now she's hooked on 5K races.

What was Meaghan reexperiencing, after more than eleven years, that compels her (like others) to continue running?

"I felt I was flying," she said simply. "Both feet were in the air at the same time."

That's precisely what's happening in joyous midstride, when both feet are airborne (whether you have two original feet or not). "My trainer had to tell me to slow down," she added. "He saw that I risked burning out."

Slowing down can be hard when you suddenly realize that you were born to fly.

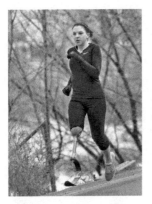

Meaghan Cusack out "flying"

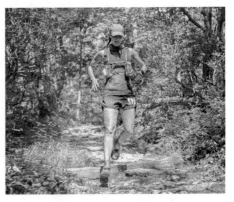

Ultra runner Sara Davidson challenges herself—and the trail.

DRILLS

Knee valgus and noncontact ACL injuries tend to occur more commonly among women. The drills related to single-leg strength, balance, and foot and hip control are foundational, and are described in other chapters:

- Single-leg stance
- Single-leg run drill
- Proper squats
- Box jumps, done correctly

Regarding nutrition, women in particular might want to note this dietary advice:

- Eat plenty of iron-rich foods (iron is lost during menstrual cycles). Red meat has the most bioavailable iron.
- Get adequate vitamin D from food and sunlight, for bone strength. Check your level. Optimal is greater than 50 ng/mL.
- Foods with vitamin K and K_2 are essential for hormonal function (quality meat, seafood, eggs, leafy greens, and full-fat dairy). Don't be afraid of high-quality organ meats, and eating "tip to tail," as traditional cultures do, and look for dark, leafy greens such as spinach, kale, chard, and broccoli. These contain fat-soluble vitamins, so they work better in combination with butter, olive oil, eggs, dairy, and meat than they do separately.
- If pregnant, you will become more prone to insulin resistance, so don't overload on simple (processed) carbohydrates. If your body is craving a certain food, you are likely missing something essential, and may benefit from consulting with a nutritionist or medical provider. Eating nutrient-poor foods rarely curbs these cravings, so chuck the junk!

- If you have any unexplained symptoms, especially if neurological, check your B_{12} status. Optimal is greater than 500 pg/mL.

And destress. As Elinor notes above, women can find a place of joy and grace in running. Talk a friend into joining you for a short run.

CHAPTER 16

Young at Heart

Our growing softness, our increasing lack of physical fitness, is a menace to our security. We do not want in the United States a nation of spectators. We want a nation of participants in the vigorous life. This is not a matter which can be settled, of course, from Washington. It is really a matter which starts with each individual family.

—PRESIDENT JOHN F. KENNEDY,
Conference on Physical Fitness of Youth, 1961

Kids today are under house arrest.

—UNKNOWN

Play as if your life depends on it.

—FRANK FORENCICH

MYTH: *Thanks to superior nutrition and training, today's youth are healthier than at any point in history.*

FACT: *Children today are a minute slower in the mile run than children of thirty years ago, and more than a third are overweight or obese.*

In America, we have built an entire culture around elite youth sports. Children and teens are groomed to excel, and selected youth are channeled into specializing in a single sport, often in order to chase the elusive goal of a college scholarship.

This parental preoccupation with excellence isn't healthy for kids. By nature, most children are motivated by a love of play, and they should be allowed and encouraged to define their own level of involvement in sports. When parents confine themselves to offering support and a place to play (and setting inspiring examples, themselves), they see better results than when they prod and push and challenge. The most significant influence on a child's level of physical activity is the parent's level of physical activity.

THERE'S NO SURE APP FOR THAT

It would seem, judging by our fascination with sporting events (and the piles of money lavished on professional teams), that American kids are fitness-crazed, and from an early age. The reality is very different. The total number of children engaged in daily exercise, formal or informal, is low and declining. In 2016 the Sports & Fitness Industry Association determined that the number of youth aged six to twelve who were active through sports on a regular basis fell to 26.6 percent—continuing a slide from 30.2 percent in 2008. The *quality* of the exercise is declining, too, such that the modest amount of exercise each child gets may not be contributing a lot to overall health.

This isn't due to lack of awareness. Most of us know that exercise is good, yet we've been gradually, insidiously sidelining regular activity for kids. Funding for physical education and fitness programs in schools has consistently been cut, and only about a quarter of children engage in physical activity outside of school. Poor nutrition, lack of recreational opportunity, and excessive computer and smartphone time all may be contributing to declining leisure time activity. The American Medical Association and other sources clearly state that decreased physical activity plays a critical role in the increase in obesity, morbidity, and chronic diseases among youth. Some observers rationalize that the incidence of obesity has plateaued in the past few years—though at a very high level. This ongoing epidemic doesn't need to be stabilized. *It needs to be reversed.* Data from 2017 unfortunately show childhood obesity is still on the rise.

A HEFTY DEFENSE CHALLENGE

Obesity and poor fitness are the biggest contributors to a startling statistic. According to 2017 Pentagon data, 24 million young Americans between the ages of seventeen and twenty-four—71 percent of the people of that age group—are ineligible to serve in the United States military. This is especially distressing when we consider President Kennedy's concern, expressed a half century ago, about the poor physical condition of the country's youth. Indeed, the first warning call was sounded in the late 1950s, when it was discovered that 58 percent of American children were unable to pass a basic fitness test. Fewer than 9 percent of Europeans failed the same test. President Eisenhower, and later Kennedy, saw the problem and took action.

Kennedy recalled that Theodore Roosevelt had required Marine officers to march fifty miles in three days, and in 1963 he challenged the commander of the Marines to see if his troops were in comparable shape to those of the early 1900s. Bobby Kennedy attracted media attention when he walked fifty miles from Great Falls to Harpers Ferry on the C&O Canal towpath—in a pair of oxfords, in freezing conditions—and made it in under eighteen hours. The fifty-mile challenge became a national craze, drawing in housewives, students, scouts, seniors, soldiers, and everyday citizens. The JFK 50 Mile was born out of this movement, and the route overlaps part of our annual Freedom's Run marathon, which starts in Harpers Ferry, West Virginia.

A STATE WITH SOME WEIGHT

Changes in diet and lifestyle have impacted not only personal performance and the conditioning of our armed forces. Increasingly, young people in general are at risk from diseases that can diminish the quality, productivity, and length of their lives. The CDC estimates that 75 percent of health care dollars are spent on chronic diseases that could be prevented. In 2011, they report, chronic diseases comprised seven of the top ten causes of death, and 86 percent of all health care spending was for people with chronic medical conditions. (End-of-life care is no small portion of this.)

For me, this situation is personal. My state of West Virginia ranks at the top in obesity, and the bottom in health programs for children. Close to 40 percent of West Virginia elementary school children are overweight or obese. And these obese children have high odds of becoming obese adults—with an 80 percent correlation in the case of obese teenagers. Insulin resistance, lifestyle, the external environment (including diet)—all tend to become more difficult to reverse as teenagers advance into their twenties and thirties. Complicating this is the role played, it is now believed, by the body's *internal* environment—the intestinal microbiome—which works to "defend" and perpetuate an obese state.

More than a third of those who were born in 2000 will be afflicted by type 2 diabetes. The current generation of youth is likely to be the first that will die at a younger age than their parents did. It's simple: children and youth of all ages need to start moving, running, and playing—especially while enjoying the outdoors. Eating well (and avoiding sugar-sweetened beverages and juices!) is essential, too, as discussed in chapter 10.

Health care providers shouldn't try to shame children into reducing body fat. Doing so can cause eating disorders and psychological damage, and generally doesn't work anyway. Exercise, healthy food, and a positive attitude—taken together in healthy doses, daily—is the best prescription for achieving a healthier body composition.

It has been understood for some time that physical activity is a key component of healthy brain development, by inducing cascades of growth factors that instruct downstream structural and functional change in the brain. A large study by Hans-Georg Kuhn and colleagues of the University of Gothenburg found that cardiovascular fitness among eighteen-year-old boys is positively associated with intelligence and educational achievements later in life, as well as with disease prevention. Exercise is fertilizer for the brain and body, and kids need more of it than do adults for optimal growth and development. Even if you disregard the *physical* health benefits of regular exercise, the boost that it gives to the brain alone should establish it as a public health priority.

We can't afford to *not* change the way people approach movement and exercise. Numerous studies show that exercise-focused public health initiatives pay substantial dividends in terms of health care savings and worker productivity. I'm working on jump-starting our state health leaders so that they can head out on this path—at a good, healthy jog.

NURTURING A PANDEMIC OF HEALTH

Speaking of paths, and in the spirit of getting kids out into nature, our nonprofit, the Eastern Area Health Education Center, is collaborating with private and public partners in our West Virginia counties to promote farmers' markets and build fitness trails at schools and parks. This is a small, local effort, and the permitting process and bureaucracy is daunting, but we're gaining ground.

First Lady Michelle Obama took one laudable step with her campaign Let's Move!, which was dedicated to eliminating obesity within one generation. The program has raised awareness, but unfortunately the youth exercise and health needle has barely budged. (In my opinion, Let's Move! didn't sufficiently focus on cutting processed and sugar-sweetened food and beverages from our diets.)

In a nationwide program I am involved in called Park Rx America, parks and medical clinics are helping reduce obesity by providing opportunities for physical activity by making it easy to search for and print out maps for local parks at clinic visits. And in our rural county, I joined a small band of citizens and school administrators to start a middle school cross-country program that took off running, so to speak, during the very first year it was offered.

The beauty of running is its simplicity. In the United Kingdom, a free, informal school program known as The Daily Mile continues to gain traction, such that half a million schoolkids are now running a mile each day during school hours. Studies have shown dramatic fitness benefits from The Daily Mile (it takes only fifteen minutes), yet when pupils were measured for academic achievement, they found scores of up to 25 percent higher in reading, writing, and math. The United States and other countries are

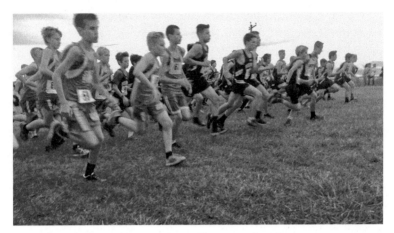

The start of the inaugural Berkeley County Middle School Cross Country Championships in West Virginia, with two hundred children participating

adopting similar programs, though at a disappointingly slow pace, thus far.

A friend and lifelong exercise physiologist, Mick Grant, describes "Fun First" as his abiding principle, and he may be on to something. In summary: *if it isn't fun, don't do it.* The corollary to this is: *stay healthy.* (If you're not healthy, it won't be fun in any case.) Whether the athlete is ten years old and runs three days a week, or eighteen years old and runs seven days a week, the goal should be *zero* days missed due to injury or illness.

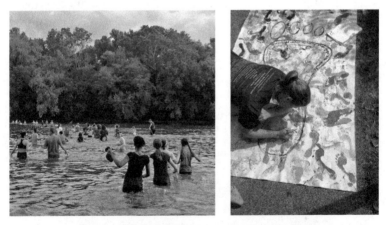

A group of middle schoolers crosses the Potomac on a run,
then prepares a canvas that illustrates why they run.

Mick also encourages kids to try different sports and activities in addition to running. Running relieves stress, and kids can talk to their friends during training runs. Proper training for running, Mick points out, demands less commitment of time than any other sport. Endurance and speed factor into most sports, and running supplements most of these, too.

The trick is to get kids to enjoy coming to practice. Athletes need to push themselves, but the process of accepting a challenge and rising to it needs to be fun. This is the philosophy that guides Mick's and my youth running initiatives.

BAREFOOT IN THE PARK

Running is one of the most accessible activities there is, and it's a superb cross-training activity for almost any competitive sport. When a child's sport isn't available to them (for instance if no field is available, if there's no team practice that day, or if they're out of town), they can always run. Throughout, it should be enjoyable, because we want kids to come back for more.

The next time you are in a park, watch a child run barefoot. Notice the relaxed movement and foot placement, and the springy body, with legs trailing out behind. When barefoot, kids don't land hard on their heels. They can change direction on a dime and never roll an ankle.

Then watch children wearing highly cushioned or supportive shoes. They look as if they've been shoehorned into hobbling prosthetic devices in order to compensate for a structural problem. All too commonly, they sprain an ankle.

Kids are naturals. Neuromuscular pathways that control form and coordination get "wired in" during childhood, and we have a tendency to develop bad habits if good ones aren't reinforced. Adults often place their kids in cushioned, confining footwear from day one. The single best intervention that parents can make on behalf of their children is to get them out of restrictive shoes and let their feet feel the earth. Free the feet!

Unfortunately, the shoe industry has succeeded at convincing parents, educators, and health care professionals that a child should wear miniature versions of traditional adult shoes—almost all of which have elevated heels, extreme cushioning, and some form of motion control technology. Cushioned shoes do not reduce injury rates among youth (and may even increase them). In the window of time before kids' feet are deformed by shoes, they still have an opportunity to walk and run naturally.

Foot specialists, too, are victims of conventional wisdom. The American Podiatric Medical Association's position paper on children's shoes cautions that the shoe should be rigid in the middle, and not twist. It goes on to add, "[This] does not apply to toddlers' shoes. For toddlers, shoes should be as flexible as possible." I wonder: at what point does a toddler become a child, and why do they suddenly need to begin binding and restricting and distorting their feet?

Let's get our kids started on the right foot. Given what we know about child development and the elements of natural running gait, here are a few things to consider before you shop for kids' shoes:

- Ultra-thin soles with no (or low) heel drop are best, *especially* for kids. This allows for good proprioception, or feel for the ground, and for neuromuscular activation throughout the entire kinetic chain. Kids learn movement and balance through proprioception, and the foot is the foundation and the messenger for that. A single-piece midsole/outsole (not two-piece) offers protection on unnatural and rough surfaces, while allowing natural dissipation of ground reaction forces.
- The shoe should be flat but bend easily at the toe joints—where the foot is designed to bend—and not impede the forming and stiffening of the arch of the foot on toe-off. The toe box should be wide enough to provide for natural outward toe spread, because the foot produces the greatest leverage when the toes are straight and aligned with the metatarsals. And look for a soft, breathable upper material that is good for repeated cycles through a washing machine, or for soaking in sports detergent (we use SweatX), with air drying. The smell

comes from bacteria (not from the dirt), and the SweatX kills it without destroying the fabric.

Kids' shoes don't need a lot of tread or traction. Shoes with stickiness and grip produce more heat and have higher braking moments (and increased torque) when running and playing, which increases the risk of sprains and tears. (This is one reason *not* to outfit a small child with cleated shoes.) Removing the sockliner insole (if the shoe has one) can improve the foot-to-ground interface, and heavy socks aren't needed, either.

Be aware of how scale affects shoe geometry and function. A 4-millimeter "drop" (differential in the elevation of the sole from heel to the ball of the foot) in a size 1 shoe has the same gradient as a 12-millimeter drop in a larger, cushioned adult shoe. Also, a 40-pound child cannot bend the midsole of a shoe that might be considered relatively flexible for a 165-pound man. The lighter the child, the more important it is that the shoe rolls up and flexes easily.

KIDS WON'T ALWAYS BE SO

Kids (and their parents) should be aware of the unsettling changes that can occur during adolescence. For natural hormonal reasons, girls' running times may be slowing. The rail-thin, springy eleven-year-old is gone in a blur, yet she often brings with her into womanhood a different body combined with an intense pressure to win. This can make her more prone to depression, injuries, and disordered eating. Healthy females lay on essential body fat during adolescence—which is a bit of a mismatch for elite distance running.

During puberty, both genders of children become susceptible to traction injuries at tendon insertion sites (and a variety of musculoskeletal syndromes) when soft tissue growth doesn't keep up with rapid lengthening of the bones. For instance, when getting into a squat, they may feel discomfort because the bones have lengthened yet the Achilles tendon hasn't kept up. Injuries can develop where the major tendons and ligaments are inserted into the bone.

Sever's and Osgood-Schlatter diseases (I prefer to call them syndromes), for instance, are typical tendinopathies at the Achilles and patellar tendon insertions that almost always resolve by the end of adolescence.

LEARN FROM THE CHILDREN

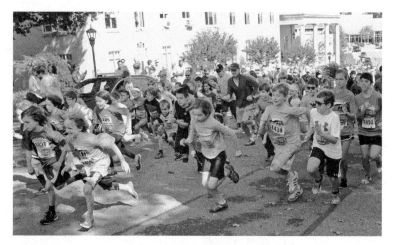

The start of the Freedom's Run kids' fun run in
Shepherdstown, West Virginia

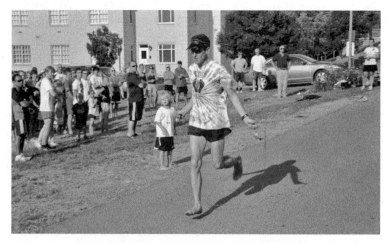

Running with a jump rope. Embrace your inner child and
rediscover movement and play!

More adults—and this includes doctors, medical researchers, and educators—need to climb into the sandbox with children. Instead, they busy themselves with crafting guidelines that no one follows. For all of us, running and movement should be approached as a form of play—the way it is for kids, who are living, fully aware, in the present moment. Running and healthy movement become sustainable for all of us only when we give ourselves permission—as kids do—to *have fun*.

DRILLS

Some favorite calisthenics for kids are linked on the videos page of the book's website, including:

- *Jump rope and jumping jacks* build rhythm and aerobic fitness.
- *Burpees.* Kids are good at these.
- *Stair hops* build strength and spring, especially in the feet, Achilles tendon, and lower leg.
- *The grapevine drill* is a simple lateral movement exercise that improves agility. This can even be done during a run.
- *Parkour.* The ultimate running play. Obstacles emerge from the terrain, and the point is to creatively navigate and utilize them, while developing your own style of smooth, efficient movement.

CHAPTER 17

Healthy at Any Age

Once, when I was a young physician, I said that the man is of the age of their arteries. Later I enjoyed writing the age of his endothelium. Today, as a retired, 84-year-old GP, I say that the age of a man is that of his mitochondria.

—SERGIO STAGNARO of Genoa, Italy,
in a comment on a *New York Times* article

Healthy life expectancy—our healthspan—*is not keeping pace with the average lifespan, and the years we spend with poor health and disabilities in old age are growing.*

—DR. ROSS POLLOCK, King's College London

MYTH: *Frailty is what happens when the body wears out, and there is little that you can do to delay this natural aging process.*

FACT: *Frailty results from not continuing to use and move and stress your body as you grow older.*

With age, we tend to lose the habit of natural, fluid movement that came to us automatically as children. But this is not an inevitable loss. Indeed, relaxed, efficient movement has been trained out of us by work (sitting), by our environment (cars and mechanical aids), and by the downright dangerous myth that we should "take it easy" when we grow old.

My dream is to see elderly people rediscover the fluid movement and biomechanics of the bodies that we were all born with. It's still there—waiting to be jump-started, revved up, and taken out on the highway. Considering that older folks come with an approaching expiration date, there's no time to lose!

EXERCISE INTELLIGENCE

It's well known that physical activity and cardiorespiratory fitness are associated with higher cognitive functioning. A study led by Agnieszka Burzynska and colleagues at the University of Illinois suggests that high-intensity physical activity has a protective effect on neural processing in aging, too. This is because exercise triggers the production of BDNF, which stimulates the growth and differentiation of new synapses and neurons, especially in areas vital to learning, memory, and higher thinking. In other words, physically fit older adults are more flexible—cognitively and in terms of brain function—than their more sedentary peers.

Diet is an actor in the aging process, too. A Stanford study found that in basically healthy people, the presence of insulin resistance is a strong predictor for a variety of age-related diseases, and for Alzheimer's in particular. ("Alzheimer's" is used generally to describe a spectrum of dementias.)

One tragic, underrecognized dimension of Alzheimer's treatment is that many patients are prescribed heavy *sedatives*. No wonder they often have blank stares. The new psychiatric medications (and a barrage of other designer drugs to address pain in Alzheimer's) that are hitting the market will do little or nothing to reverse dementia.

Movement and exercise, on the other hand, *can* improve it, noticeably if not significantly. Dementia specialist Dr. Dale Bredesen and colleagues have demonstrated success with a novel, personalized therapeutic protocol originally known as MEND (metabolic enhancement for neurodegeneration), and now called ReCODE (Reversal of Cognitive Decline). His model for "patching 30 holes in the roof" combines exercise with an anti-inflammatory and low-glycemic diet, good sleep, hormone and micronutrient optimization, MCT oils, and even a touch of red wine. The ReCODE protocol, when followed, has helped patients recover enough to return to work.

The good news is that more people will live into their eighties than ever before. The bad news is that the odds of dementia at age eighty-five are 50 percent. Plaques and tangles in the brain are presumed to be the primary indicators of Alzheimer's, although half of patients who present with the clinical spectrum of Alzheimer's don't have them. Healthy elderly people can exhibit substantial plaque and tangles, which to some extent are present in normal aging.

There's more to the Alzheimer's story. Our brains are remarkably neuroplastic, and we are wired to develop work-arounds. The more we use a movement, the more that movement becomes available to us. PET scans are one encouraging diagnostic tool: they are superior to MRIs for illuminating brain activity, and for assessing the variety of pathologies that can appear as Alzheimer's.

Insulin resistance that occurs in the brain itself is referred to as type 3 diabetes. This happens when high glucose levels (and corresponding hyperinsulinemia) trigger "glycation" of brain proteins, along with inflammatory responses that damage nerves. Neuropathy is an expected complication of poorly controlled diabetes. Central neuropathy (dementia) is the worst kind. Faulty aging might suitably be termed "inflamaging."

RUNNING INTO OLD AGE

So, will running help you to live longer? Despite some scares in the media that running is dangerous, the answer is *yes*—at least the majority of the evidence points that way. As sports medicine pioneer Dr. Gabe Mirkin says, "The only mechanism ever found to prolong life and delay aging is exercise. There is no data whatever to show that antioxidants, vitamins, or anything else prolongs life." This is partly because when you take supplements and antioxidants, you don't get the "training effect"—meaning your body isn't stimulated to produce these substances on its own.

Our aerobic strength declines as we age. But not necessarily by much. In what's familiarly called the Dallas Bedrest and Training

Study, five healthy twenty-year-old male college students were subjected to three weeks of strict bed rest. Before and after their confinement to leisure, researchers measured their VO_2 max—the standard metric for exercise capacity, and a good indicator of one's "physical" age. At the end of the three-week period, the students' average VO_2 max declined by 27 percent. (Afterward, they engaged in an eight-week exercise program that restored their original fitness, and then some.)

The surprise came when the same subjects were studied thirty years later. Over the intervening three decades of living reasonably healthy and active lives, their average VO_2 max declined *less* (from the first pretest baseline) *than it had during their three weeks of bed rest.* I've conducted many treadmill tests and measured VO_2 max in patients and runners myself, and I see fit seventy-year-olds who score younger than out-of-shape twenty-year-olds. This doesn't mean, of course, that the decline due to aging is fully preventable. It does mean that we can stay active, healthy, and strong until late in life.

LIFE SPAN ≠ HEALTH SPAN

Medical science counts our modern-day gain in life expectancy, and the statistical decline in age-adjusted death rates, as victories. Longevity—the *quantity* of our lives—has increased slightly in recent years, yet we haven't seen a corresponding extension in the *quality* of our lives. Nowadays, a higher percentage of us are reaching advanced ages—over eighty, for instance—but it isn't clear whether, on average, our *functional* life spans are longer than they were decades ago.

Natural selection does a pretty good—not perfect—job of weeding out the unhealthy. All of us are the descendants of winners in natural selection. Take a look at your family tree, back to your grandparents' generation or earlier. Find a truly healthy ancestor— one who lived into their nineties. In all likelihood, they were active and healthy until reasonably close to their time of death. How did they live, and what did they eat?

In my experience, most active people don't exercise to increase

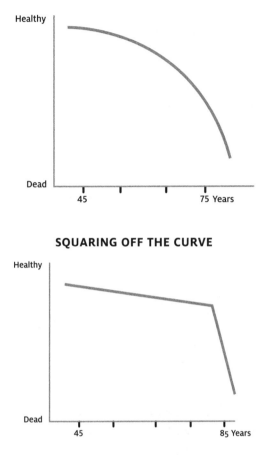

CURVE OF MODERN AGING

SQUARING OFF THE CURVE

The graph on the top describes the slow decline typical of modern Americans as they age. But it's entirely possible, with healthful living, to follow the path on the bottom. Dr. Ken Cooper (the author of *Aerobics*) coined the phrase "squaring off the curve."

their longevity anyway. They simply sense that they live better and fuller lives when they do.

In an article in *Biogerontology* called "Live Strong and Prosper," researcher Michael McLeod and his team confirm that aging is accompanied by a slowing in the growth of skeletal muscle, and a decline in muscle mass (sarcopenia). These factors are directly associated with mortality in the elderly, largely because they place them at greater risk for falls.

Physician and author Walter Bortz asked a pertinent question: *What comes first, frailty or sarcopenia?* When you confine an elderly person with a narrow margin of strength in bed, it's very difficult for them to *ever* emerge and reclaim full health. The goal of the patient (hopefully supported by their care provider) should be to remain upright and mobile, as long as possible. By increasing muscle protein synthesis, through activity and exercise, a strong, healthy muscle mass can be maintained. This greatly improves functionality and independence, reducing the chance of injury from a fall.

Orthopedist Dr. Vonda Wright has also demonstrated sarcopenia in the MRIs below, images from two people in their seventies. The one on the bottom (the more physically active one) shows double the amount of muscle as the one on the top, though their body weights are roughly equal.

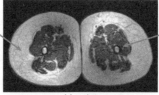

ADIPOSE TISSUE   QUADRICEPS

70-year-old sedentary man

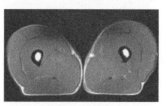

74-year-old triathlete

One study found that only two weeks of limitations on walking (in an otherwise free-living condition) resulted in decreases in insulin sensitivity, lean leg mass, and VO_2 max. We need to be vigilant. The risk of becoming diabetic (if you aren't already) increases as you age and suffer extended downtime.

A GENUINE, SELF-GENERATED FOUNTAIN OF YOUTH

When we age, we typically face a variety of degenerative diseases. Contrary to conventional wisdom, running can help alleviate these by promoting *healthful* stresses, which in turn trigger cellular regeneration and even neurogenesis. The body is constantly repairing and growing, turning over cells—almost completely replacing them every eighteen months. This turnover is like replacing a gigantic girder bridge one section at a time while keeping the bridge open. The destiny of machines is to "use it *and* lose it"— they wear out. But for biological organisms such as our bodies, it is "use it *or* lose it." We have a choice.

We want the functional use to continue, of course, and hopefully we can even enhance it. It's easy: if we apply good food, love, enjoyment, and movement, then positive growth and repair will occur naturally, even when we are older.

GOING OVER A HUNDRED, PEDAL TO THE TRACTOR METAL

Frank Buckles was the last surviving World War I veteran in the United States. (He also spent four years in an internment camp in Italy during World War II.) After an enjoyable evening with his family, he died peacefully at the age of 110.

Frank was a neighbor of mine. During the period that he lived in rural West Virginia until the day of his death, he scrupulously observed three rules of good health:

1. *You must stress the body.*
2. *Never be in a hurry.*
3. *Don't worry.*

He did morning calisthenics into his nineties, including standing on his head. He slowed down only when a piece of farm equipment dented his skull, which made it difficult for him to maintain his balance. He drove his tractor until he was 103 (you can imagine his response when doctors suggested, years earlier, that he was too old to climb onto it), and he continued to work on the farm until he was 105. Occasionally, after prodding from friends and family, Frank would see a physician. But the physicians inevitably prescribed meds, and Frank dumped them in the trash almost every time. The one drug he did take for aches and arthritis (not surprising at 110 years) was an occasional ibuprofen.

I believe that Frank developed an extremely efficient metabolic system during his time at a civilian internment camp in Italy, when he was given one cup a day of food. He had the self-control to divide the cup into thirds and eat portions throughout the day. Some studies have linked dietary restriction to a slowed aging process, though this is difficult to test and prove.

Genetics plays a role in how you age, but *how you live* is a larger factor—and it's within our control, after all. Considering our busy, high-stress culture, *Don't worry* is perhaps Frank's most overlooked piece of advice. Stress hormones routinely flood through our veins as a physiological response to the numerous psychological challenges that greet us nearly every day.

The Mayo Clinic cautions that the stress response is activated so often in many of us that the body may not have adequate opportunities to return to normal, leading to a state of chronic stress (indicated by prolonged high bloodstream levels of cortisol, the "stress hormone"). Chronic stress impairs cognitive performance, suppresses thyroid function, and causes blood sugar imbalances (such as hyperglycemia), decreased bone density, decrease in muscle tissue, elevated blood pressure, lower immunity, slowed wound healing, and inflammatory responses throughout the body.

That sounds a lot like what we see in aging.

Persistent high levels of cortisol also boost the buildup of adipose tissue—belly fat—which is linked to even more serious health problems: heart attack, stroke, metabolic syndrome, and higher levels of the damaging, small-particle-sized low-density lipoprotein.

To keep cortisol levels under control, the body's relaxation (parasympathetic) response should be activated promptly following a fight-or-flight (sympathetic) response. Frank Buckles's secret was that following incidents of stress, he could quickly reset his parasympathetic system at healthy levels and reclaim a relaxed, clear mind. This topic is covered in chapter 13, and is especially applicable as we grow older.

TRAVELING BY FRAIL ROAD

These days, elderly patients are spending a shorter time living and a longer time dying.

Among elderly patients, I see a lot of frailty. The first thing I do is have them stand up from a sitting position. If they have difficulty, I work with them on the mechanics of standing, by helping them find their center of gravity and adjusting their posture and form. I also observe their walking speed. Slow walking speed is associated with multiple poor health outcomes.

Although a solid medical definition of frailty is elusive, it refers to the phase of life when we lose our independence and our health. Many assume that frailty is the inevitable result of wearing out our bodies and minds. In fact, it comes from lack of use. As soon as you stop using your body, the decay and decline timepiece starts ticking. As Walter Bortz put it, "The body is like a grandfather clock: every day you have to wind it up."

And not just wind up the body. Cranking up the mind and keeping it invested with tasks, direction, and meaning is a critical part of the package, too. Longevity, we're coming to understand, isn't just physical. It's associated with *a feeling of purpose* and with *a connection to community*. Isolation is associated with accelerated aging.

Most important, we should remain positive and not worry about things we *used* to be able to do without effort. Rather, focus on what we *can* do, enjoy doing it, and look to the future for all that is new. As Abraham Lincoln said, "I may walk slow, but I don't walk backwards."

Every day, I try to pause for a moment and consider Frank Buckles's three simple rules for health. He showed me that aging well is a true endurance sport.

OH, YEAH—OA

Osteoarthritis is the leading cause of disability among the elderly, and it affects as many as a quarter of us when we reach the age of fifty-five.

Many people believe that running is injurious to joints. It's true that running and other impact sports, when done improperly, can increase the risk of knee trauma and osteoarthritis in the knee. But Paul Williams and colleagues at the Lawrence Berkeley National Laboratory found that even for recreational runners who participate in multiple marathons annually, running does not appear to increase osteoarthritis and hip replacement risk. For one thing, running can help control body weight, which is a risk factor for osteoarthritis. But running may even offer *protection* from osteoarthritis, by promoting cartilage thickening and by enhancing its viscoelastic properties. Walking, and low-impact exercise such as biking, Williams found, offer no particular protective advantage.

YOUNGER NEXT YEAR

The medical literature on aging guides us to a simple conclusion: *stay active and keep moving.* Those whose lives are characterized by prolonged sitting tend to acquire disease, including dementia, and become frail at an earlier age than nonsitters and regular exercisers. Once you become sedentary, the decay process is set in motion, and it doesn't matter if your blood pressure and other health lab indicators are "within normal limits." Once you're bedridden, frankly, it's all downhill from there.

The *Journal of the American College of Cardiology* compares physical activity to a miracle drug. "The list of diseases that exercise can prevent, delay, modify progression of, or improve outcomes for, is longer than we currently realize." One research team found that running as little as five to ten minutes per day was associated with a 30 percent reduction in mortality from all causes, a 45 percent reduction in mortality from cardiovascular disease, and an addition of three years to life expectancy. The benefits of exercise for healthy aging can compensate for some of obesity's negative impact on aging.

For many of us, visits to a clinic or hospital comprise the rare moments when we are faced with (sometimes uncomfortable) medical reality. If we want to grow old, it's best to start preparing now, before that clinic visit. Being sedentary and overweight alone doesn't normally send us to the doctor, though as we age its implications for health, longevity, and vulnerability to disease are clear and serious.

The Hippocratic Oath requires that doctors "first, do no harm." In my view, this *obliges* us to discuss the health effects of obesity and physical inactivity. If doctors and the medical establishment don't proactively raise these issues with patients—which usually entails addressing their lifestyles—we are doing a disservice to them and to our profession.

Insurance reimbursements focus on treatment. Physicians have little financial incentive to recommend preventive exercise and lifestyle changes. Additionally, many of them may not even know what physical activity to prescribe, nor where to send their patients. I feel that they *must* summon the best sources of knowledge and experience that they can. By educating themselves, they will be positioned to motivate their patients and our society, and to abandon old habits, wishful thinking, and symptomatic treatment. We'll all appreciate it when we're older.

DRILLS

Aging readers can begin by "resetting" their bodies every day, by working on posture and balance, and by keeping the fascia supple. How to do this? Start by kicking off your shoes. Make yourself tall, and stretch out like a cat. Find your balance and your connection with the ground.

It may sound rudimentary, but work on *properly arising from a chair*, especially when you are weak from bed rest or an ailment:

1. Position yourself in a seat, not too high or too low, with thighs parallel to the floor.
2. Scoot your butt forward and tuck your feet under your hips; maintain a wide stance (the width of your hips).
3. Lean forward (as if being tugged from the sternum), pivoting from the hips, and stand up in a single, fluid motion.
4. Stand up in this manner two or three times every half hour—then gradually increase the frequency.

A lab test that aging readers might like to consider (be careful what you ask for!) is a telomere length test. Your telomeres are the dynamic, protective caps on the ends of your DNA strands. Healthy, long telomeres reflect healthy cell replication and remodeling, and they tend to shorten with age. I was relieved that my results showed me as a (gratefully) much younger man—thirty-five in "telo years"—despite my busy and stressful life.

CHAPTER 18

The Nature Cure

In every walk with nature, one receives far more than he seeks.
—JOHN MUIR

In many modern societies, biophilia and the recognition of nature's extensive values [lie] dormant. Our present day context of sprawling settlements, enslaving technology, compulsive consumption, and weak natural sciences educational curriculums account for much of this disconnection and apathy, and yet at significant socio-economic and potentially irreversible environmental costs.
—HELEN SANTIAGO FINK

MYTH: *Exercise promotes health, regardless of where you are.*

FACT: *Evidence shows that physical activity in nature provides additional levels of mental and physical health and well-being.*

Nature is something we tend to forget, or take for granted, yet it ties much of this book together. The natural world is the source of the food we eat, the air we breathe, the water we drink, and the resources that go into the products we consume. Evidence strongly suggests that exposure to nature benefits physical and mental health in a variety of important ways, and can derail disease before it develops.

Humans are a species—highly evolved, we believe—that is inextricably linked to the natural world. And by moving our bodies through the range of motion we were designed for, including running, we become an extension of nature. What could be more fulfilling than to express ourselves in the most complete and natural way we can? And what more appropriate place to use and care for our bodies than in the environment in which we evolved? Medical researchers understand much about what happens to us physiologically when we exercise. We know less about the more intangible qualitative benefits of moving and *being* in the outdoors.

Sports, which are generally done outside, are a proxy for managing the challenges of nature. It may be no coincidence that some of the most popular *individual* sports are those that place the human body in a natural setting with only minimal tools or mediation: mountaineering, rock climbing, skiing, surfing, and swimming. And running. These activities pivot around the same basic goal: *to efficiently and gracefully negotiate the challenging terrain ahead, assisted by little more than the bodies and minds we were born with.* (Or, from another perspective, to simply get through it without falling, crashing, or sinking.)

AN EPIDEMIC OF E-DEVICES

The average number of hours per day that people spend indoors on digital devices seems only to climb, while our time spent outdoors—and in nature, especially—declines. Children and "screenagers" are especially vulnerable to a physically nondemanding but attention-robbing indoor lifestyle, such that we are broadly witnessing what Richard Louv (author of *Last Child in the Woods*) has termed "nature deficit disorder." The habit of remaining indoors continues even as we learn how interior, manufactured environments (along with the poor nutrition and lack of physical activity that tend to accompany them) contribute to obesity, high blood pressure, type 2 diabetes, heart disease, depression, and many other illnesses.

It's as if kids these days are under self-imposed (or parent-directed) house arrest. A study by Frances Kuo and colleagues found that children who engage in outdoor activities in nature exhibit significantly fewer symptoms of attention deficit hyperactivity disorder (ADHD) than children who engage in activities in other settings. These findings were consistent across age, gender, and income groups, as well as geographic regions and diagnoses. Related research has shown that children with ADHD focus better on tasks after as little as only twenty minutes outdoors. Outdoor play in natural environments also fosters improved relationships among children and better cooperation, communication skills, and creativity.

The mental health benefits from time spent in nature may even exceed the significant physical benefits. Experiments performed by Marc Berman and researchers at the University of Michigan have demonstrated nature's broad restorative value in terms of cognitive functioning. "Nature, which is filled with intriguing stimuli," he concludes, "modestly grabs attention in a bottom-up fashion, allowing top-down, directed-attention abilities a chance to replenish." Urban environments, by contrast, overflow with stimuli that continually demand our top-down attention (to avoid being hit by a car, for instance, or to continually check that your handbag is safe). This ultimately depletes rather than restores cognitive function.

In another study, Ruth Ann Atchley and colleagues confirmed that exposure to nature can replenish our ability to focus attention on a specific task. Atchley sent fifty-six women (who had never previously hiked) out into a remote area for four days, disconnected from all media and technology. Before their hike, they were tested on creative problem-solving tasks that draw upon higher-order cognitive skills. Four days later—while still out in nature—they were tested again. Their performance improved by 50 percent.

WHEN IT COMES TO THINKING, LESS IS MORE

In addition to a short-term performance boost on cognitive tasks, exposure to nature may offer longer-term benefits to mental well-being. A study by Gregory Bratman and colleagues at Stanford compared participants who went on a ninety-minute walk through a natural environment with those who walked through an urban environment. The nature walkers reported lower levels of rumination—repetitive, self-referential, negative thoughts—and showed increased neural activity in the subgenual prefrontal cortex. Deactivation of this area of the brain is linked to an increased risk of depression and mental illness.

More than half of the world's population now live in urban areas, and by 2050 this proportion will reach 70 percent. Bratman's findings suggest that in our rapidly urbanizing world, investments in access to natural environments could yield valuable mental health dividends for urban dwellers.

A PRESCRIPTION WITH ENDLESS FREE REFILLS

Although "nature deficit disorder" isn't recognized as a medical term, I hope that it will gain broader currency, applying to a variety of physical, mental, and emotional symptoms that correlate with isolation from the natural world and lack of exposure to sunlight.

Family physicians are especially well positioned to treat it. As doctors, it behooves us to help connect our patients, especially youth, to the outdoors—for the same reasons that we need to initiate more doctor-patient conversations about prediabetes, diet, and obesity.

I'm honored to be a part of several collaborations with government agencies, corporations, physicians, and local civic groups. Nature Prescriptions is one of these, and we are dedicated to improving public health by linking the health care system to our public lands. Especially useful are the maps and info on regional parks and trails. (The *Discover the Forest* page, for example, includes a park finder that is searchable by zip code.)

The National Environmental Education Foundation is another organization that has zeroed in on getting kids more involved with nature. And the Children & Nature Network, cofounded by Richard Louv, is dedicated to getting kids, families, and communities reconnected to the natural world.

FILL THIS PRESCRIPTION IN YOUR LOCAL FOREST

Motivated by the objective of improving public health, even the National Park Service has gotten in on the act. The national Park

Rx initiative (parkrxamerica.org) is a coalition of health providers, public land agencies, national nonprofits, community organizations, and the NPS, offering park prescriptions programs across the nation. (Yogi Bear takes on a whole new meaning.) And Park Rx America helps doctors to offer their patients access to a free health resource—their local parks. A patient's electronic medical record shows their zip code, and doctors can offer patients a map of their local parks and trail systems. Currently, the network draws from an online database of more than 350 green spaces in the D.C. area, now expanding to a wider region, including West Virginia. The receptionist prints out the patient's local map as they depart.

If you're located in an urban area, a city park is better than no park. Some may argue that urban green spaces, while pleasant, don't offer much of a dose of unmitigated nature. But they provide valuable respite and restoration from chaotic urban life. City parks not only boost individual health and mental wellness, but they are good for the cities, too, due to the cooling effect of evaporation from soil, grass, trees, and waterways. Urban green spaces also offset the absorption of heat by concrete and asphalt. Buildings located around parks use less energy for cooling.

Jennifer Wolch and colleagues found that among three thousand children aged nine and ten, those with access to parks (within five hundred yards) and recreation programs (within six miles) had a significantly reduced risk of obesity at age eighteen. And simply painting urban spaces green brings people outside more often.

You cannot medicate your way to health. Medications and therapy are marginally effective for many chronic conditions. As a doctor, I feel it is essential to prescribe nature to most of my patients. (If only nature prescriptions could be billed to insurance companies, more doctors and medical professionals would prescribe them.) Why do many medical doctors—clinical biologists, in effect—seem to view and treat humans as separate from the natural, biological world? Too often, what physicians see and treat are diseases of captivity.

With my patients, I usually approach the topic indirectly. Rather than ask, for instance, "What do you do for exercise?" I'll say, "What do you like to do that involves movement outdoors?" Continuing in this vein, I might ask, "How does it make you feel when you come back from that activity?" or "How do you feel if you've gone a week without getting outside or visiting a park or natural area? Do you prefer to be solitary, or with a group, and move with intensity, or in a leisurely way?"

How a patient feels is not a bad indicator of their health. So I solicit a bit of subjective medical history by asking, "During what period of life did you feel the best?" and then have them tell me *why* that is. The process of simply sharing this information serves to remind them of the value of the activity.

As a follow-up, I'll ask, "Would you like to find a way to do more of that?" Then I might offer some background on the benefits of walking, for instance, especially if the patient has high blood pressure or insulin resistance. In a way, I'm prescribing *purpose:* a means to reach a level of vitality that will make them feel better.

I give patients permission—okay, I encourage them—to go outside in almost any conditions and circumstances. As a medical student working for the Alaska Native Health Service, I lived in Nome for three months in the dead of winter and saw little sunlight. As often as I could, I went out and ran on the firmly packed Iditarod Trail. The cold, blustery weather was refreshing and rejuvenating, and it woke up not only my mitochondria and capillaries, but also my entire nervous system. (I started my runs into the wind, so that I could save the homeward, downwind leg as a reward at the end.)

People have somehow been convinced that the environment for exercise needs to be comfortable and homogeneous. I don't recall enjoying running any less in Nome than I do now that I'm back in a much warmer climate. The body needs to experience a variety of environments in order to adapt and thrive. Look at the conditions that wild animals endure, and the adaptations they make. They can survive extremes of heat and cold, throttle up intensity (such as when chasing prey or running from predators), and sleep or hibernate (when they need to conserve energy). Like our animal kin, we evolved to function well in many circumstances and all seasons. To replicate that, we should add new and different stresses each day. There's no bad weather, it's said—there's only bad clothing (and lassitude). If you're like me, the most memorable experiences transpire when conditions are unfavorable.

RUNNING OFF INTO THE WOODS

I have a number of colleagues and friends who are committed, athletic runners, yet they've never entered a road race. They are trail running enthusiasts. In addition to a refreshing shot of nature, trails offer the challenge and stimulation of changing terrain, and they generate less impact than hard pavement.

One friend, Bill Susa, began running in 1996, at age thirty-four. The same year, he was diagnosed with a cardiac arrhythmia. Less than a month later his father—an avid and accomplished runner—died.

"You would think that would be it for me," Bill told me, "but I was convinced I had to stick with running—not only as a touchstone to my father, but for my own physical health." In 2005, he moved to within a mile of the Appalachian Trail, and discovered trail running. "I have been hooked ever since," he said. "It's my chapel, my meditation, and my source of inner peace. It has helped me through a nasty divorce, estrangement from my daughter, and the high stresses of my career—I'm an air traffic controller."

Then in 2014, Bill was diagnosed with adrenal fatigue, attributed mainly to disruption of his circadian rhythms from his erratic work routine. "Between working different shifts every day of the week and trying to train seventy to ninety miles a week, I was on an unsustainable trajectory."

Bill couldn't *not* run. So he took a break and dialed back his training mileage (and performance expectations), and normalized his work schedule. After a few months he began making progress toward recovery. Along the way, he changed his point of view.

"Now, I'm saddled with—or enlightened by—a new reality. I view my trail runs not in terms of training, but as a form of recovery that is spiritually, physically, and emotionally necessary for my overall well-being. On each run, I await that magical, transcendental moment when my conscious mind shuts down and I find myself floating effortlessly down the trail, one with my surroundings. Each leaf, each stone, each tree becomes a part of me, and I an equal part of them. As the trees whiz by, I feel the tethers that bind me to my health challenges slip away. My mind enters what I can best describe as a state of flow. Brain chatter—good, bad, and indifferent—ceases, and in that moment, in that span of immeasurable time, I'm enshrouded not by my limitations, but by a wellspring of hope: *I am free, and alive.* This is what I imagine heaven feels like."

SEEKING OUT NATURE SURPLUS SYNDROME

I haven't met anyone who seriously tried trail running and then gave it up. Nearly everyone who gets into it stays into it. I believe that's because trail runners think not in terms of *having* to go out and run, but *getting* to. As good as indoor cardio classes can be, I'm not sure they muster the same motivation, nor offer the same rejuvenating thrill and enjoyment, of trail running.

So get off your computer, get outside, get active, and make your feet your friends! The celestial realm that Bill Susa found in nature awaits.

DRILLS

- *Head for the sun!* Bask in the robust body of evidence that the sun and fresh air generate positive hormonal and mental effects. Healthy, restful sleep is essential on the far end of the daily spectrum—and this is boosted heartily by time you spend outdoors on the near end.

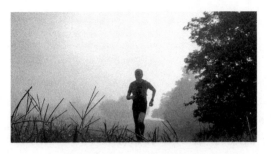

- *Get a dog,* or spend time with the one you have. Dogs know what's best for you—hence their insistence that you walk or run or move outside. Their companionship mitigates the isolation that is often a by-product of the modern, digital world.
- *Take a trip into nature.* Go hiking or even car camping. You'll find that your mind (and priorities) "reset," and that your awareness, focus, cognitive abilities, and feeling of well-being will return with you to civilization. The Japanese call this forest bathing.

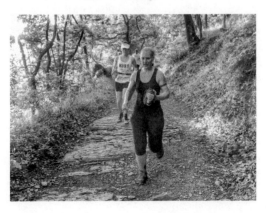

CHAPTER 19

Running in Place:
The Health of Our Communities

*This knowledge, the knowledge that the physical well-being
of the citizen is an important foundation for the vigor and
vitality of all the activities of the nation, is as old as Western
civilization itself. But it is a knowledge which today, in
America, we are in danger of forgetting.*

—PRESIDENT JOHN F. KENNEDY

MYTH: *Running is a lonely, solitary pursuit, primarily offering
a sense of personal accomplishment.*

FACT: *Running is more about health and mental well-
being—a big part of which comes from connection,
community, and sharing.*

President Kennedy's words were spoken more than a half century
ago, but his exhortation is yet to be fully heeded. The average level
of physical fitness in America, which many considered low in 1962,
has not declined. At the same time, right in front of our eyes, our
attention is being outsourced to digital screens, retail megachains,
and corporate monopolies. (It's discouraging, when I'm running
in a new neighborhood and ask for directions, to typically hear,
"Take a right at the Burger King, then a left at the Applebee's . . .")
Even homegrown events such as running races are increasingly
managed by companies that charge high entry fees and leave
behind large environmental footprints—with little involvement of

the locally rooted, personally invested, joyously connected culture of family, friends, and neighbors.

It's time to take back our communities.

IT'S BEST IF YOU CAN STAY AWAY FROM US . . .

As a physician, I'm keenly aware that the *medical community,* too, needs to step out of the hospitals and reach into our neighborhoods and backyards. We need to be accountable to the needs of the people we serve, and treat patients as members of a healthy community, not as victims of diseases. Through evolution, an organism changes and adapts in order to survive and thrive. It's time for the medical community to evolve.

This may sound self-evident, but the *three-trillion-dollar* (annual) health care industry in the United States is a bit of a mess. Reimbursement is based on the *quantity* of treatment we deliver—in the form of tests, visits, procedures, drugs, devices, and other interventions—while health care providers, policy makers, insurance companies, and interest groups are left to haggle over who will pay the ever-rising costs. It's like a city with an abundance of auto diagnostic and body repair shops but no driving schools.

Our disease-based health care system has devolved into a complex, disjointed, expensive, and sometimes dangerous mix of medications, specialists, shifting payers, and complex rules. The term "preventive care" has been invoked so much that it has become a cliché. It implies that better health is dependent on the *care* (such as screenings and exams) of a health provider. But true prevention means making an effort to stay away from us. As Max Planck said, "Science advances one funeral at a time."

Our ritual of the annual physical exam, for instance, has *not* been shown to save lives, improve health, or decrease costs, at the same time that accepted screening tests such as colonoscopies, PSAs, Pap smears, cholesterol checks, and even mammograms are blunt tools at best. At worst, when applied broadly to healthy populations, these tests can result in more tests, and costly and painful interventions.

By some measures, yes, Americans are living longer than they did a hundred years ago. But in many cases they are paying a price for this by *becoming unhealthier at an earlier age*. Type 2 diabetes, high blood pressure, and other chronic conditions are becoming pediatric conditions, and the pool of those afflicted is becoming larger. In the *Military Times*'s recent report that 70 percent of high school students are ineligible for military service, "insufficient health and fitness" was the primary reason. In order to maintain needed recruitment levels, the military is debating now whether to further lower the fitness bar.

CULTIVATING HEALTH

As both an athlete and a physician, I feel that this business of health needs more consideration and thinking, and less treatment. Many athletic injuries are best treated by physical therapists, coaches, friends, and oneself (plus a bit of time), rather than by doctors. As Ben Franklin said, "God heals, and the doctor takes the fees."

Many of these treatments and therapies, and their astronomically high costs, could be avoided if we invested more thought into *how we live*. Specifically, that means more attention needs to be paid to policies and programs that support active, healthy lifestyles for people of all ages. Researcher Chi-Pang Wen and colleagues advocate the building of *a culture of physical activity*. Although most patients are aware of the benefits of daily exercise, the researchers conclude, "It is up to us to move them from wishful thinking to a practical reality." Public health happens in the community, not in the doctor's office.

GLOBAL COLD SPOTS FOR HEALTH

The benefits of a healthy lifestyle are undeniable. Several carefully controlled longitudinal studies have shown that in the aggregate, long-living people from cultures around the globe share a number of healthy practices and daily habits. These populations, in what are referred to as global health "cold spots," share something else, too: when they emigrate and adopt modern lifestyles and diets, they quickly become as unhealthy as the residents of their adopted homes. So it's not a matter of genetics.

There is nothing new or revolutionary about healthy, traditional lifestyles. Indigenous groups engage in moderate physical activity throughout their lives, eat a varied (mostly whole food) diet, maintain their weight, don't smoke, and live in communities that *give care* forever. The elderly are woven into the cultural fabric, and they continue to provide service and value as they age. They're not abandoned to the mercy of a corps of paid caretakers and medical providers. And—gratefully—no one tells them to relax and take it easy.

A perfect example is Clarice Morant, who died at 104. After the age of 100, she bathed and fed two aging family members in her own home. As Clarice *gave care,* she received life and health in return. This is true prevention, and real community.

FAMILY JOGGING, KIWI STYLE

Some communities have successfully worked together to improve their collective health and well-being. The idea of family "jogs," for instance, was developed in New Zealand in the 1950s by the legendary coach Arthur Lydiard, who founded the Auckland Joggers Club, which included many cardiac patients. (The idea that heart patients should jog, which is now a standard of care, was wildly controversial at the time in America.) Lydiard's Sunday-morning gatherings of young and old, walkers and joggers (and a few serious runners), turned into a weekly, block-party-like tradition across New Zealand.

In 1962, the legendary University of Oregon running coach (and cofounder of Nike) Bill Bowerman traveled to New Zealand to observe Lydiard's coaching techniques for Olympic-level athletes. But it was the broader jogging sensation that most struck him, and when he returned to Oregon he began hosting Friday-evening jogs. At first, a handful of adventurous souls gathered. Soon hundreds appeared. Today, the city of Eugene is widely recognized for its network of trails, community health initiatives, and culture of outdoor recreation.

SPREADING JOY AROUND THE BLOCK

Those who see running as painful drudgery—or as an occasional tedious, hard-won victory—may find it hard to turn around and envision it as an abiding source of joy. So how do we change that perception and make running fun for large numbers of people? How do we take the next step and use running as a means of reclaiming the health of our communities?

As individuals, we can begin by slowing down our movements and our thoughts and merely experience the marvelous complexity of the body as it moves through space—seeing our own selves, and those around us, as functional works of art. Much of that beauty lies in the simple, joyful act of *maintenance*—housekeeping for the body—that takes the form of daily movement.

We can, as we run, remind ourselves that running is also about connection. Jogging, vigorous activity, team sports, running races, and combined effort toward a common goal—all of these forge bonds with friends and companions that remain for life. I haven't heard of a single medical school lecture on the topic of *community*, but the World Health Organization counts it as one of the leading "Determinants of Health." The corollary is also true: social isolation can be as injurious to one's health and longevity as smoking is.

Many folks in my home state of West Virginia aren't known to be optimal specimens of health, and I don't think many of them look upon running as a source of joy. The rest of the country isn't doing much better. The developed world has become a culture without movement—or aspires to be—and much of the developing world is following this lead. Too many of us share the goal of *avoiding* exercise and unnecessary activity, and we've largely reached that goal by successfully engineering much of the movement out of our lives. (For our decades of hard work and technological advances, after all, haven't we earned some rest and comfort?)

Sure, professional sports are huge—at least the business of sports is. For the players, however, it has become the reserve of an elite band of gladiators. Excellence is tied to punishing, hard-to-attain goals that don't always coincide with overall health for the athletes, and certainly not for the spectators.

FREEDOM'S RUN—A TRUE COMMUNITY EVENT

In 2009, my community of Shepherdstown, West Virginia, set out to change that. I began to offer medical seminars, running workshops, community fun runs, and (with a dedicated band of fellow volunteers) large running events. Throughout, we've been motivated by the simple desire to see folks get outside and start enjoying physical activity—and bring their friends and family along for the ride. Healthy living is not a spectator sport.

This effort has birthed Freedom's Run: An Event for Health and Heritage—an annual citizens' fun run that has triggered a shift in our local culture by reconnecting children and families to nature and fitness. The event has generated a snowball of local business sponsors for the race, and their employees show up to run and to volunteer. Everyone is welcome to enter the one-mile fun run, 5K, 10K, half marathon, or marathon, and each year more than twenty-five hundred participants from at least forty states join in. The tenth annual Freedom's Run will be held in 2018, and it's the biggest running event in West Virginia.

Through osmosis and word of mouth—the best form of outreach—this fun run concept has spread to other communities. The Freedom's Run team has been lending support to growing numbers of regional events, and the eastern panhandle of West Virginia now hosts more than twenty running races each year (up from only four, nine years ago). Also local, the Harpers Ferry Half Marathon (which I co-direct) is headed into its tenth year, too. And a large community running group called "Bros and Bras," born at the 2014 Freedom's Run, now has more than four hundred active members. (Their motto is "No judgment, no expectations.")

Freedom's Run has raised over $200,000 for local health, history, and heritage initiatives. We have partnered in funding twelve school-based fitness trails, a 2.4-mile trail around a new county park, and a program called Canal Classrooms, which brings fourth graders from West Virginia and Maryland to the C&O Canal Visitor Center in Williamsport for a day of outdoor, place-based learning.

The best part of these running races is that people from cities and distant locales get to experience an organically homegrown

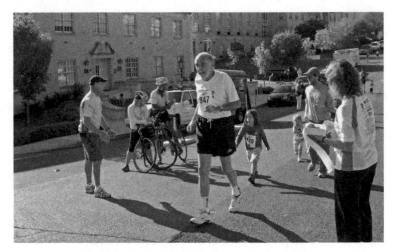

The old and young run together at Freedom's Run.

event in a small, cohesive community. The courses take runners (and walkers) through Harpers Ferry National Historical Park, the C&O Canal National Historical Park, along the Potomac and Shenandoah Rivers, and through Antietam National Battlefield. Entrants say they feel invigorated simultaneously by nature, history, and camaraderie. (Visit the Freedom's Run home page at freedomsrun.org. And to get a feel for how this event impacts our community—and a glimpse of one of our first community fun runs—view the short videos at runforyourlifebook.com.)

Most important, all of these events, races, and running groups are fashioned around a spirit of collaboration—a convergence of kids, socializing, connection, and community well-being. Participants share a feeling that we're all in it together, that together we can reclaim our fit, healthy lives.

A WHOLE NEW "FARMACEUTICAL" INDUSTRY

In 1960, the average per capita amount spent on health care was *one-third* the amount spent on food. This situation has more than reversed, such that in 2015 America spent $10,340 per person on health care—*more than double* what they spent on food (and that includes eating out in restaurants). As a share of personal income, Americans now spend less on food than does any other country in the world.

Might there be a link between cheap food and escalating health care costs? The seriousness and prevalence of diabetes alone requires that we persist in asking this question, and in evaluating all of the available evidence. The cost of care for a type 2 diabetes patient has reached a staggering, unsustainable level of almost $20,000 per year.

I'm convinced that every additional dollar that individuals spend on *healthful* food saves us many multiples of dollars in downstream public and private health care costs. Indeed, the medical care we offer in West Virginia and the subsequent health outcomes depend, at a basic level, on our patients' ability to buy healthful foods.

The West Virginia University School of Medicine and Health Sciences Center is on a trajectory to become a center of excellence for physical activity, nutrition, and healthy lifestyles. In 2017 we opened the Center for Diabetes and Metabolic Health, where I'm focusing on low-carbohydrate nutrition. We are also reaching into the heart of rural West Virginia and introducing folks to the health benefits of the "farmacy"—the abundance of natural, unprocessed, healthy foods from local farms.

In partnership with the USDA and nonprofits such as Wholesome Wave and the Benedum Foundation, WVU is helping Supplemental Nutrition Assistance Program (SNAP) recipients make their money go further at participating farmers' markets. (Shockingly, the most common purchase made by SNAP recipients is sugar-sweetened beverages.)

Through what's called the West Virginia FresHealthy Bucks program, when SNAP recipients swipe their EBT cards to purchase vegetables, meat, eggs, and other farm staples, they are given *double* that value in the form of FresHealthy Bucks, the currency that can be used only at the farmers' market. The difference is made up by WVU and the partners when the vendors are reimbursed at the end of the day.

The FresHealthy Bucks program not only helps the individuals it serves but also gives a boost to the local farmers and farmers' markets—a true bootstrapping operation! Going into its fourth year, in 2018, the program generated more than $25,000 in SNAP-supported business.

Our next task is to scale this up.

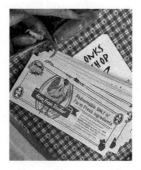

FresHealthy Bucks, redeemable at local farmers' markets

A SMALL STORE WITH A BIG (BUT MINIMAL) FOOTPRINT

I also feel lucky to be able to contribute to our community through a small, nonfranchise running store I own called Two Rivers Treads, which focuses on teaching healthy running. In defiance of conventional business models, as the nation's first minimalist shoe store we strive to sell customers *less* running shoe—while demonstrating that it's possible to survive and thrive in the age of big-box stores. We do this by paying near-obsessive attention to customer service. Visitors to Two Rivers Treads undergo an evaluation in which my staff and I help them understand the way their body moves, and sometimes reinvent the way they run. In 2016, Two Rivers Treads was recognized by *Competitor* magazine, and by the Independent Running Retail Association, as one of the top fifty running stores in the country. I attribute this to our dedication to the community and to public service.

It's satisfying to get people out running, but seeing the Two Rivers Treads employees succeed is my greatest reward. Serving customers is enjoyable work, but I don't expect all the young staff to work in a running shoe store forever. Two have graduated from physical therapy school, and two are at U.S. military academies. Another qualified for the Olympic Trials for track and field in 2016, and is now a contender for the 2020 Olympic team.

THE END IS THE BEGINNING

The running races, the healthy food programs, the community outreach—and the shared exhilaration of effort and movement—are small but important ingredients in the recipe for restoring public health. Through self-reliance and dependence on one another (rather than on professionals or the Internet), we can help rebuild a culture of community and sharing. One by one, we can initiate this by joining a tribe of like-minded joggers, hikers, or whatever—any group whose members share a passion for movement, activity, and health.

Our modern culture is drifting away from nature, from our original way of being, and we're suffering the physical and mental consequences. I'm convinced that the global community awaits a *Silent Spring* type of awakening in the realms of medicine, health, agriculture, nature, and community self-reliance. It's my dream that—someday, together—we can teach ourselves how to train, to eat well, to prevent and manage injuries, and to extend the functional length of our lives. Perhaps we can even live up to President Kennedy's hope that all of us, by leading lives of vigor, will create a healthy America. We're in a race with no finish line.

It may sound paradoxical, but I feel that the goal of this book will be reached when you *don't* have to think about the principles and the drills described here. This eventuality will come when you have fully integrated its contents into your daily life—your movement, your work, and your relaxed state of mind. And ultimately, it's not about the running. It's about the merging of body, soul, and community into a healthy way of being.

DRILLS

- Get out and run with friends, relatives, or folks in your neighborhood.
- Organize a group run or race—for any number between two and two thousand people.
- Volunteer at a race, a food bank, a community kitchen, or as a mentor for kids in your community.
- Find a sense of purpose in your community, and in social connectivity with others. The health-sustaining effects of this extend beyond the spectrum of medical indicators.
- Find purpose to all that you do, because cultivating a vision and goal sets the stage for productivity and happiness. I'm eager to go to work every day, pursuing my goal of helping people find a healthy path forward. Purpose is my most important prescription.

Appendix I

WEB RESOURCES

Please visit the *Run for Your Life* website, runforyourlifebook.com, to view the videos (/videos) and find additional resources. Direct links to most of the drills and other resources referred to in this book are provided through this single web portal, where you will find, organized by chapter, a menu of:

- Smartphone- and laptop-viewable videos of drills—including posture, exercises, and running form.
- Links to articles, blogs, training modules, lectures, reviews, demonstrations, and other resources and references. In particular, some links will take you to my collection of resource materials at Dr. Mark's Natural Running Center site (http://naturalrunningcenter.com), Dr. Mark's Desk (drmarksdesk.com), and Two Rivers Treads (tworiverstreads.com).

Appendix II

DRILLS FOR A LIFETIME

I am sometimes asked to provide a rigorous, progressive training schedule that runners and active people can dutifully execute and adhere to. For those who want to reach for a specific running goal, such as entering a 5K, 10K, half marathon, or marathon, appendix III offers tried-and-true training regimens, structured around running itself.

The drills summarized in *this* appendix, which are meant to improve movement and strength, are more open-ended and self-directed. In my experience, most of us—who aren't on a competitive training schedule—simply aren't very dutiful or diligent about following a cumbersome list of drills. If an exercise or movement doesn't feel good or provide a feeling that it is helping us, we tend to stop doing it. Like the act of running itself, the drills we do must be fun and safe, and make us feel better.

I have only one strict demand of my readers: get up off the couch, get outside, and move. And when you find the movements and the drills that work for you—your favorites—just keep doing them. I do recommend that you experiment with all, or most, of the drills in this book. Try them. In the process, (1) you will learn about how your body works and feels, where your tight spots are, and where your posture or position is out of whack. And (2) you will be able to identify the drills and movements that feel good, that suit you, and that address your shortfalls in neuromuscular control.

In summary, make a note of the drills and movements that work best for you. Then keep doing them.

Most important, jump (!) at every opportunity you can to interrupt your sedentary habits and move your body—as vigorously as feels comfortable—through its full range of motion. Garden. Help someone move. Walk or ride a bike instead of driving. Do lunges. Whenever you can, take stairs two at a time. At meetings and public events, stand up at the back or along the wall. Claim and covet the most physically demanding tasks for yourself. Someone's needed to crawl into tight spaces, carry the groceries, sit on the floor, or run back for a dropped glove? That's for you. The musician Meat Loaf said it best: "There ain't no Coupe de Ville hiding at the bottom of a Cracker Jack box."

The drills in this book are as much for beginners as they are for veteran athletes and marathon runners. If you're new to running, out of shape, or not especially athletic, just begin slowly and easily. Stay within your comfort zone. As strength and endurance build—which they will—you'll find that more repetitions, with greater intensity, and with a greater range of motion, will come naturally and pleasurably. More speed and power is the *result,* not the *goal.*

The drills and exercises distilled here—my own favorites—can be done at your own pace, gauged to the level of exertion and difficulty that suits you. Personally, I try to incorporate several drills in my daily workouts, or as "exercise snacks" while at work or at home. I select the exercises according to my mood, to the amount of time I have, and to my specific areas of weakness. I mix it up, and always engage the drills with a sense of play.

Perform *your* favorite drills at least a few times a week, for about ten minutes. It's best to do these on days when you are not fatigued, and after you are warmed up. Less, done correctly, is better than more, done incorrectly.

I've distilled these drills into four groups: "Mostability," "Awakening your springs," "Strengthening your springs," and "Extras." The summaries of them here are referenced to page numbers in the text, for more complete descriptions. Also, I urge you to see the *Run for Your Life* website (runforyourlifebook.com) for videos of most of the drills that are listed here.

MOSTABILITY (MOBILITY AND STABILITY)

You're up, mobile, outside (or in the gym)—and ready to move. That means you're most of the way there! Do these movements throughout the day and you will be more prepared to run consistently and without injury. I do short versions of these when I am warming up before a run, too. We know that forceful stretching is not beneficial before running, but many of these movements are "dynamic" stretches, because you are increasing your mobility and releasing restrictions through *controlled, gentle movement—not* by pulling and stretching.

TRY THESE POSITIONS OR DRILLS:	Video reference
Short foot posture. This is your foundation. Train the foot throughout the day, as you stand and walk.	Short Foot
Single-leg balance. Single-leg stability is key. Master this for thirty seconds with eyes opened, and fifteen seconds with eyes closed. (If you can, move into a single-leg hop and run, described later.)	Single Leg
Golfer's pickup. Bend at the waist as if picking up a golf ball—swinging one straight leg directly behind you, while keeping the balancing leg straight.	Golfer's Pickup
Leg swings. Stand tall, keep your pelvis neutral and stable, and swing your leg like a pendulum—forward and back, and side to side.	Leg Swings
Lunge matrix. Focus on balance and smoothness.	Lunge Matrix

TRY THESE POSITIONS OR DRILLS:	Video reference
Mountain climber. Done correctly, this is great for opening the hips.	Mountain Climbers
Awesomizer. This can be done any time you can place your foot on a chair or stool. It involves balance, rotation, hip extension, and an upper body reset, all in a smooth movement.	Awesomizer
Supple hips. The supple hips/windshield wiper progression is my morning hip opener. It maintains internal and external hip rotation. Great for your golf swing, too.	Supple Hips
Six-position foot walk. A perfect exercise snack.	Six-Position Foot Walk
Heel raises. While balancing on your right foot, slowly lift your heel so that you are balancing on the ball of your foot. Switch feet.	Heel Raises
Mindful walking. Pay attention to an erect posture, smoothness of movement, and efficiency. Press off the big toe. Get your arms moving and upper body rotating—feel the spring as your stride opens up behind you.	Mindful Walking
Backward walking. This works the muscles on the back of the leg. Keeping the thigh vertical, bend the knee so that the shin is horizontal. Make sure you know where you are going.	Backward Walking
Abdominal breathing. Breathe slowly and deeply, pulling your diaphragm toward your spine as you exhale.	Abdominal Breathing

AWAKENING YOUR SPRINGS

Even if you are fit and healthy, you may well have lost that pop off the ground that is so critical for running. Let's start by restoring this—by waking up our springs.

TRY THESE POSITIONS OR DRILLS:	Video reference
Light hopping, and skipping rope. Jumping rope builds elastic recoil. This trains our feet and ankles to work like powerful springs. Jump with light, quick, full-foot contact, timed to a cadence of about 180 beats per minute. When your cadence, springiness, and rhythm are good, add the jump rope. Start with a duration of one minute, and build to five minutes. Then try running with it.	Jump Rope
Ninja squat jumps. Begin by doing a few to a low platform the height of a curb. Focus on landing softly, with low impact. Raise the platform gradually. Practice jumping down, also quietly.	Ninja Squat Jumps
Experimental barefoot jogging. Try it for short distances, slowly, on clean pavement. It will remind you of good running technique: smooth, with low impact.	Barefoot Jogging

STRENGTHENING YOUR SPRINGS

Now that you have a little spring in your step, you can add a few more challenges (in a safe and low-intensity way). Proceed cautiously, and avoid anything painful. Good mechanics and fast, springy feet are the goals. Never do these drills to the point of fatigue or failure.

TRY THESE POSITIONS OR DRILLS:	Video reference
Burpees. Doing sets of six to eight of this age-old exercise is safe, fun, and sustainable.	Burpees
The grapevine drill (also known as karaoke). Moving sideways, keep your arms outstretched, and have the trailing leg alternately go across the front, then the back. Keep the upper body still while the hips rotate through 180 degrees.	Grapevine
Strides, or pickups. In the middle of your run or after your run, two or three days a week, do ten-second sprints: turn it on, lengthen your stride, and test your full range of motion.	Strides
Lateral jumps. Jumping sideways, with feet together, is a great skiing exercise and recruits your lateral hip stabilizers. Stand alongside any type of object from one inch to mid-shin height—a log, for instance. Jump over it, back and forth, for ten reps, staying on the ground as little as possible. Aim for three or four sets.	Lateral Jumps

TRY THESE POSITIONS OR DRILLS:	Video reference
Single-leg hop/run. After mastering the single-leg balance, become a one-legged pogo stick and hop on one foot, with minimal ground contact time. Then try running a short distance on one leg.	Single-Leg Run
Run with a tether. Run while restrained by a stretchy tether (and while standing on a mini-trampoline, if available). Maintain a neutral posture as you focus on driving away from the anchor.	Run with Tether
Turkish getup. The perfect full-body strengthening excercise	Turkish Getup

EXTRAS

There are a handful of additional, highly beneficial drills that are best demonstrated by live people, and are not included in the text. Please visit the videos page of the *Run for Your Life* website (runforyourlifebook.com) to see these excellent drills performed.

TRY THESE POSITIONS OR DRILLS:	Video reference
World's greatest stretch and sumo. After the lunge matrix, there is no better progression than these two multiplanar, dynamic movements. Together, they open up not just your lower extremities and hips but also your torso and shoulders.	World's Greatest Stretch and Sumo
The heel lift drill. This teaches us to lift the foot by using the back of the leg, instead of the front, by activating the glutes and hamstrings. While doing this, lean slightly forward (or backward), as if on a Segway. The goal is to maintain springy contact with the ground, not to run fast.	Heel Lift
Ankling, or fast feet. Fold your foot elastically down to the surface, from toe to heel. The heel barely touches the surface before bouncing off, as you push down and back from the glutes. Keep the cadence high. Relax your upper body, and move your feet—fast!	Fast Feet
Stair or curb hops. With a sense of play, move up and down on a stair (or curb). Land softly and quietly as you step up and step down, lightly hopping. Focus on quick, springy, and quiet feet. Begin slowly!	Curb Hops

TRY THESE POSITIONS OR DRILLS:	Video reference
Four square. Like hopscotch. Do a single-leg hop, with quick direction changes, in a square pattern. Make a square grid on the floor with tape, do it on a tile floor to simulate the grid, or simply eyeball your marks on the ground.	Four Square

ABCD skips. Become a sprinter again, and relearn this classic track drill.
 	
    A SKIPS: with strong hip extension, propel yourself forward with a high knee flight.
 	
    B SKIPS: pull the leg down with the glutes and hamstrings, preparing for the impact phase.
 	
    C SKIPS: extend from the push-off leg, like a ballet leap. Keep the pelvis neutral.
 	
    D SKIPS: with a strong and springy foot, flick the heel up toward the glutes.
 	
Perform these in a series, A-B-C-D, traveling forward about 10 yards each time. Then relax, turn around, and return to the start with a fast 40-meter stride. Do four to six sets of these, making sure to fully recover between sets.
	ABCD

123 run. A simple progression to start a run with proper technique	123 Run
Principles of natural running. At a million views and going strong, learn the basics of natural running	Principles of Natural Running

TRY THESE POSITIONS OR DRILLS:	Video reference
Barefoot running style. My first barefoot running video, presented at the 2011 Boston Marathon.	Barefoot Running Style
Going for a run. One of life's simple pleasures is going for a run outside.	
West Virginia kids running revolution. Kids are our future.	WV Kids Run Revolution

This may appear to be an ambitious, or even daunting, list of drills. Simply do the ones that feel right, and when you are done be sure to include the most important drill of all: chill out—relax and recover. Breathe deeply, walk mindfully, eat healthfully, and sleep well.

Appendix III

TRAINING PLANS FOR A 5K, A HALF MARATHON, AND A MARATHON

If you would like to work up to competition—even for a modest goal such as a citizens' 5K race—then you may benefit by adopting the training plans that follow. As always, you should count on progressing slowly, in sequence, as you build endurance and strength. The path to competition is not a race.

The first of these training schedules, "To 5K and beyond," is designed for the runner who is just starting out, or returning to running after an extended break, or recovering from illness or injury. The goal throughout is to develop a safe and gradual adaption to fitness.

It's not essential that you follow these schedules rigidly. The matrices are flexible, and include a variety of activities, so that you'll make movement a daily—and fun—habit. If you are already partially fit, you can pick up this schedule somewhere in the middle. But be honest with yourself. Listen to your body.

By the final weeks of the sixteen-week "To 5K and beyond" plan, you should be comfortably jogging for thirty minutes, most days of the week. *Only then embark on the half-marathon (twelve-week) or marathon (sixteen-week) plans once you have developed the aerobic system.*

Unlike with some other training regimens, here I emphasize aerobic development, running skills, mobility, strength, stability, enjoyment, play, long-term progression, and overall health—*not* high-intensity workouts. High-intensity training programs can offer short-term gains, but at a high risk of injury, and often declining overall health. There is no risk with aerobic development.

Most important, pay attention to recovery, which is the time when you actually gain fitness and health. Nutrition, rest, and destressing are critical. As Dr. Tim Noakes reiterates, "What you are training for is to live a long and productive life, and maintain health." This was repeatedly confirmed, from long experience, by the legendary Arthur Lydiard when he said, "Train, don't strain."

Make activity a daily habit, and you'll succeed in both fitness and in health.

TO 5K AND BEYOND—SIXTEEN-WEEK TRAINING PLAN

■ speed/endurance ◆ running strength/quickness

	MONDAY	TUESDAY	WEDNESDAY
	Aerobic	Recovery	Long/aerobic
1	❤ 15–20 min: Walk	Rest or ✖ 30 min:	❤ 15–20 min: Walk ● Strength
2	❤ 20–25 min: Walk ◆ Drills	Rest or ✖ 30 min:	❤ 20–25 min: Walk ● Strength
3	❤ 5 min: Walk then 1 min/5 min: Run/walk intervals X 5 ◆ Drills	Rest or ✖ 30 min:	❤ 5 min: Walk then 1 min/5 min: Run/walk intervals X 5 ● Strength
4	❤ 5 min: Walk then 1 min/4 min: Run/walk intervals X 6 ◆ Drills	Rest or ✖ 30 min:	❤ 5 min: Walk then 1 min/4 min: Run/walk intervals X 6 ● Strength
5	❤ 5 min: Walk then 2 min/3 min: Run/walk intervals X 8 ◆ Drills	Rest or ✖ 30 min:	❤ 5 min: Walk then 2 min/3 min: Run/walk intervals X 10 ● Strength
6	❤ 5 min: Walk then 2 min/2 min: Run/walk intervals X 10 ◆ Drills	Rest or ✖ 30 min:	❤ 5 min: Walk then 2 min/2 min: Run/walk intervals X 10 ◆ Strides ● Strength
7	❤ 5 min: Walk then 3 min/2 min: Run/walk intervals X 7 ◆ Drills	Rest or ✖ 30 min:	❤ 5 min: Walk then 3 min/2 min: Run/walk intervals X 7 ◆ Strides ● Strength

❤ aerobic development   ✖ cross-training (fill in the blank)   ● strength training

THURSDAY	FRIDAY	SATURDAY	SUNDAY
Recovery	Aerobic	Tempo or long run	Recovery
Rest or ✖ 30 min: _____	❤ 15–20 min: Walk	❤ 15–20 min: Walk or ✖ 30 min: _____	Rest or fun active play
Rest or ✖ 30 min: _____	❤ 20–25 min: Walk ◆ Drills	❤ 20–25 min: Walk or ✖ 30 min: _____ ● Strength	Rest or fun active play
Rest or ✖ 30 min: _____	❤ 5 min: Walk then 1 min/5 min: Run/walk intervals X 5 ◆ Drills	❤ 5 min: Walk then 1 min/5 min: Run/walk intervals X 6 ● Strength	Rest or fun active play
Rest or ✖ 30 min: _____	❤ 5 min: Walk then 1 min/4 min: Run/walk intervals X 6 ◆ Drills	❤ Maximum aerobic function test: 2–3 miles ● Strength	Rest or fun active play
Rest or ✖ 30 min: _____	❤ 5 min: Walk then 2 min/2 min: Run/walk intervals X 10 ◆ Drills	❤ 5 min: Walk then 2 min/2 min: Run/walk intervals X 12 ● Strength	Rest or fun active play
Rest or ✖ 30 min: _____	❤ 5 min: Walk then 2 min/1 min: Run/walk intervals X 10 ◆ Drills	❤ 5 min: Walk then 2 min/1 min: Run/walk intervals X 12 ● Strength	Rest or fun active play
Rest or ✖ 30 min: _____	❤ 5 min: Walk then 3 min/1 min: Run/walk intervals X 8 ◆ Drills	❤ 5 min: Walk then 3 min/1 min: Run/walk intervals X 10 ● Strength	Rest or fun active play

	MONDAY Aerobic	TUESDAY Recovery	WEDNESDAY Long/aerobic
8	♥ 5 min: Walk then 4 min/2 min: Run/walk intervals X 8 ♦ Drills	Rest or ♥ 15–20 min: Jog or ✖ 30 min: _____	♥ 5 min: Walk then 4 min/2 min: Run/walk intervals X 6 easy hills ♦ Strides ● Strength
9	♥ 5 min: Walk then 4 min/2 min: Run/walk intervals X 8 ♦ Drills	Rest or ♥ 15–20 min: Jog or ✖ 30 min: _____	♥ 5 min: Walk then 4 min/1 min: Run/walk intervals X 8 easy hills ♦ Strides ● Strength
10	♥ 30 min: Aerobic run 3 min/2 min: Run/walk intervals X 7 ♦ Drills	Rest or ♥ 15–20 min: Jog or ✖ 30 min: _____	♥ 5 min: Walk then 5 min/2 min: Run/walk intervals X 6 easy hills ♦ Strides ● Strength
11	♥ 35 min: Aerobic run ♦ Drills	Rest or ♥ 15–20 min: Jog or ✖ 30 min: _____	♥ 5 min: Walk then 6 min/2 min: Run/walk intervals X 6 easy hills ♦ Strides ● Strength
12	♥ 35 min: Aerobic run ♦ Drills or ■ Time trial attrack: 1.5 miles	Rest or ♥ 15–20 min: Jog or ✖ 30 min: _____	♥ 5 min: Walk then 6 min/1 min: Run/walk intervals X 7 easy hills ♦ Strides ● Strength
13	♥ 35 min: Aerobic run ♦ Drills	Rest or ♥ 15–20 min: Jog or ✖ 30 min: _____	■ 5 min: Walk then 7 min/1 min: Run/walk intervals X 6 hills or fartlek ♦ Strides ● Strength

THURSDAY	FRIDAY	SATURDAY	SUNDAY
Recovery	Aerobic	Tempo or long run	Recovery
Rest or ♥ 15–20 min: jog or ✖ 30 min:	♥ 5 min: Walk then 4 min/1 min: Run/walk intervals X 8 ◆ Drills	♥ Maximum aerobic function test: 2–3 miles ● Strength	Rest or fun active play
Rest or ♥ 15–20 min: Jog or ✖ 30 min:	♥ 5 min: Walk then 4 min/1 min: Walk/run intervals X 8 ◆ Drills	♥ 5 min: Walk then 4 min/1 min: Walk/run intervals X 12 ● Strength	Rest or fun active play
Rest or ♥ 15–20 min: Jog or ✖ 30 min:	♥ 5 min: Walk then 6 min/1 min: Run/walk intervals X 6 ◆ Drills	♥ 5 min: Walk then 6 min/1 min: Run/walk intervals X 8 ● Strength	Rest or fun active play
Rest or ♥ 15–20 min: Jog or ✖ 30 min:	♥ 5 min: Walk then 6 min/1 min: Run/walk intervals X 6 ◆ Drills	♥ 5 min: Walk then 8 min/1 min: Run/walk intervals X 7 ● Strength	Rest or fun active play
Rest or ♥ 15–20 min: Jog or ✖ 30 min:	♥ 5 min: Walk then 10 min/1 min: Run/walk intervals X 3 ◆ Drills	MAFT 2–3 miles	Rest or fun active play
Rest or ♥ 15–20 min: Jog or ✖ 30 min:	♥ 5 min: Walk then 15 min/1 min: Run/walk intervals X 3 ◆ Drills	♥ 5 min: Walk then 20 min/2 min: Run/walk intervals X 1 15 min/2 min: Run/walk intervals X 2 10 min/2 min: Run/walk intervals X 1 ● Strength	Rest or fun active play

	MONDAY	TUESDAY	WEDNESDAY
	Aerobic	Recovery	Long/aerobic
14	❤ 35–40 min: Aerobic run ◆ Drills	Rest or ❤ 15–20 min: Jog or ✖ 30 min: _____	■ 5 min: Walk then 8 min/1 min: Run/walk intervals X 5 hills or fartlek ◆ Strides ● Strength
15	❤ 40 min: Aerobic run ◆ Drills	Rest or ❤ 15–20 min: Jog or ✖ 30 min: _____	❤ 40 min: Aerobic run ◆ Strides pickups ● Strength
16	❤ 40 min: Aerobic run ◆ Drills	Rest or ❤ 15–20 min: Jog or ✖ 30 min: _____	❤ 40 min: Aerobic run easy hills ◆ Strides ● Strength

THURSDAY	FRIDAY	SATURDAY	SUNDAY
Recovery	Aerobic	Tempo or long run	Recovery
Rest or ♥ 15–20 min: Jog or ✖ 30 min: _____	♥ 5 min: Walk then 20 min/2 min: Run/jogintervals X 2 ◆ Drills	♥ 5 min: Walk then 20 min/2 min: Run/walk intervals X 1 15 min/1 min: Run/walk intervals X 2 ● Strength	Rest or fun active play
Rest or ♥ 15–20 min: Jog or ✖ 30 min: _____	♥ 40 min: Jog ◆ Drills	♥ 5 min: Walk then 30 min/2 min: Run/walk intervals X 1 20 min/2 min: Run/walk intervals X 1 10 min/2 min: Run/walk intervals X 1 ● Strength	Rest or fun active play
Rest or ♥ 15–20 min: Jog or ✖ 30 min: _____	♥ 40 min: Aerobic run ◆ Drills	Rest or fun active play	**Run a 5k!**

HALF MARATHON—12-WEEK TRAINING PLAN

■ speed/endurance   ◆ running strength/quickness

	MONDAY	TUESDAY	WEDNESDAY
	Hills, intervals, or fartlek	Recovery	Long/aerobic
1	*Be sure to warm up by walking and jogging before all speed and endurance workouts.* ■ 5 min intervals X 3 1–2 min walk/jog between intervals Goal: 2 miles at 10K pace ◆ Drills and/or strides	❤ 20–30 min: Jog or ✖ 30 min: ――――― ● Strength	❤ 30–40 min: Aerobic run including 3 to 4 mile MAFT during run ◆ Strides
2	■ 30 min: Fartlek or hill run ◆ Drills and/or strides	❤ 20–30 min: Jog or ✖ 30 min: ――――― ● Strength	❤ 40–45 min: Aerobic run ◆ Strides
3	■ 45 min: Hilly run *Quicker on the uphills. Practice opening your stride, increasing turnover and relaxing legs on the downhills.* ◆ Drills and/or strides	❤ 20–30 min: Jog or ✖ 30 min: ――――― ● Strength	❤ 40–45 min: Aerobic run ◆ Strides
4	■ 4 min intervals X 4 1–2 min walk/jog between intervals Goal: 2–3 miles at 10K pace ◆ Drills and/or strides	❤ 20–30 min: Jog or ✖ 30 min: ――――― ● Strength	❤ 45–50 min: Aerobic run including 3 to 4 mile MAFT ◆ Strides
5	■ 45 min: Fartlek or hill run ◆ Drills and/or strides	❤ 20–30 min: Jog or ✖ 30 min: ――――― ● Strength	❤ 50–55 min: Aerobic run ◆ Strides

❤ aerobic development ✖ cross-training (fill in the blank) ● strength training

THURSDAY	FRIDAY	SATURDAY	SUNDAY
Recovery	Aerobic	Tempo or long run	Recovery
❤ 20–30 min: Jog or ✖ 30 min: _____ ● Strength	❤ 40 min: Jog ◆ Drills	❤ 60 min: Long run	Rest or fun active play
❤ 20–30 min: Jog or ✖ 30 min: _____ ● Strength	❤ 40 min: Jog ◆ Drills	■ 40 min: Tempo run *Go out easy, finish fast and strong* ◆ Drills and/or strides	Rest or fun active play
❤ 20–30 min: Jog or ✖ 30 min: _____ ● Strength	❤ 40 min: Jog ◆ Drills	❤ 60–70 min: Long run	Rest or fun active play
❤ 20–30 min: Jog or ✖ 30 min: _____ ● Strength	❤ 45 min: Jog ◆ Drills	■ 50 min: Tempo run *Go out easy, finish fast and strong* ◆ Drills and/or strides	Rest or fun active play
❤ 20–30 min: Jog or ✖ 30 min: _____ ● Strength	❤ 45 min: Jog ◆ Drills	❤ 80 min: Long run	Rest or fun active play

	MONDAY	TUESDAY	WEDNESDAY
	Hills, intervals, or fartlek	Recovery	Long/aerobic
6	▉ 50 min: Fartlek or hill run ◆ Drills and/or strides	❤ 20–30 min: Jog or ✖ 30 min: _____ ● Strength	❤ 40–45 min: Aerobic run ◆ Strides

7	▉ 5–6 min intervals X 4
	  1–2 min walk/jog between intervals
	  Goal: approx. 3 miles at 10K pace
	◆ Drills and/or strides
		❤ 20–30 min: Jog or
		✖ 30 min:
		
		_____
		● Strength
			❤ 50–55 min: Aerobic run
			◆ Strides

8	▉ 40–45 min: Fartlek or hill run ◆ Drills and/or strides	❤ 20–30 min: Jog or ✖ 30 min: _____ ● Strength	❤ 60 min: Aerobic run including 3 to 4 mile MAFT ◆ Strides

9	▉ 5–6 min intervals X 4
	  1–2 min walk/jog between intervals
	  Goal: approx. 3 miles at 10K pace
	◆ Drills and/or strides
		❤ 20–30 min: Jog or
		✖ 30 min:
		
		_____
		● Strength
			❤ 75 min: Aerobic run
			◆ Strides

10	▉ 45–50 min: Fartlek or hill run ◆ Drills and/or strides	❤ 20–30 min: Jog or ✖ 30 min: _____ ● Strength	❤ 70 min: Aerobic run ◆ Strides
11	▉ 45–50 min: Fartlek or hill run ◆ Drills and/or strides	❤ 20–30 min: Jog or ✖ 30 min: _____ ● Strength	❤ 45–50 min: Aerobic run including 3 to 4 mile MAFT ◆ Strides

12	▉ 4 min intervals X 3
	  2–3 min walk/jog between intervals
	  Stay relaxed, keeping some speed in taper
	◆ Drills and/or strides
		❤ 20–30 min: Jog or
		✖ 30 min:
		
		_____
		● Strength
			❤ 30 min: Aerobic run
			◆ Strides

THURSDAY	FRIDAY	SATURDAY	SUNDAY
Recovery	Aerobic	Tempo or long run	Recovery
♥ 20–30 min: Jog or ✖ 30 min: ⬤ Strength	♥ 45 min: Jog ◆ Drills	⬛ 55 min: Tempo run *Go out easy, finish fast and strong* ◆ Drills and/or strides	Rest or fun active play
♥ 20–30 min: Jog or ✖ 30 min: ⬤ Strength	♥ 50 min: Jog ◆ Drills	♥ 90 min: Long run *Try to cover 8–9 miles comfortably. Use walk breaks if needed.*	Rest or fun active play
♥ 20–30 min: Jog or ✖ 30 min: ⬤ Strength	♥ 50 min: Jog ◆ Drills	♥ 90 min: Long run *Try to cover 9–10 miles comfortably. Use walk breaks if needed.*	Rest or fun active play
♥ 20–30 min: Jog or ✖ 30 min: ⬤ Strength	♥ 50 min: Jog ◆ Drills	⬛ 55 min: Tempo run *Go out easy, finish fast and strong* ◆ Drills and/or strides	Rest or fun active play
♥ 20–30 min: Jog or ✖ 30 min: ⬤ Strength	♥ 50 min: Jog ◆ Drills	♥ 90 min: Long run *Try to cover 9–10 miles comfortably. Use walk breaks if needed.*	Rest or fun active play
♥ 20–30 min: Jog or ✖ 30 min: ⬤ Strength	♥ 50–60 min: Jog ◆ Drills	⬛ 55 min: Tempo run *Go out easy, finish fast and strong* ◆ Drills and/or strides	Rest or fun active play
Rest	♥ 50–60 min: Jog ◆ Drills	Rest	⬛ **Half-marathon day!**

MARATHON—16-WEEK TRAINING PLAN

■ speed/endurance　　◆ running strength/quickness

	MONDAY	TUESDAY	WEDNESDAY
	Hills, intervals, or fartlek	Recovery	Long/aerobic
1	*Be sure to warm up by walking and jogging before all speed and endurance workouts.* ■ 5 min intervals X 3 　1–2 min walk/jog between intervals 　Goal: 2 miles at 10K pace ◆ Drills and/or strides	♥ 20–30 min: Jog or ✖ 30 min: —————— ● Strength	♥ 30–40 min: Aerobic run including 3 to 4 mile MAFT during run ◆ Strides
2	■ 30 min: Fartlek or hill run ◆ Drills and/or strides	♥ 20–30 min: Jog or ✖ 30 min: —————— ● Strength	♥ 40–45 min: Aerobic run ◆ Strides
3	■ 45 min: Hilly run *Quicker on the uphills. Practice opening your stride, increasing turnover and relaxing legs on the downhills.* ◆ Drills and/or strides	♥ 20–30 min: Jog or ✖ 30 min: —————— ● Strength	♥ 40–45 min: Aerobic run ◆ Strides
4	■ 4 min intervals X 4 　1–2 min walk/jog between intervals 　Goal: 2–3 miles at 10K pace ◆ Drills and/or strides	♥ 20–30 min: Jog or ✖ 30 min: —————— ● Strength	♥ 45–50 min: Aerobic run including 3 to 4 mile MAFT ◆ Strides
5	■ 45 min: Fartlek or hill run ◆ Drills and/or strides	♥ 20–30 min: Jog or ✖ 30 min: —————— ● Strength	♥ 50–55 min: Aerobic run ◆ Strides

❤ aerobic development   ✖ cross-training (fill in the blank)   ● strength training

THURSDAY	FRIDAY	SATURDAY	SUNDAY
Recovery	Aerobic	Tempo or long run	Recovery
❤ 20–30 min: Jog or ✖ 30 min: _____ ● Strength	❤ 40 min: Jog ◆ Drills	❤ 60 min: Long run	Rest or fun active play
❤ 20–30 min: Jog or ✖ 30 min: _____ ● Strength	❤ 40 min: Jog ◆ Drills	■ 40 min: Tempo run *Go out easy, finish fast and strong*	Rest or fun active play
❤ 20–30 min: Jog or ✖ 30 min: _____ ● Strength	❤ 40 min: Jog ◆ Drills	❤ 60–70 min: Long run	Rest or fun active play
❤ 20–30 min: Jog or ✖ 30 min: _____ ● Strength	❤ 45 min: Jog ◆ Drills	■ 50 min: Tempo run *Go out easy, finish fast and strong* ◆ Drills and/or strides	Rest or fun active play
❤ 20–30 min: Jog or ✖ 30 min: _____ ● Strength	❤ 45 min: Jog ◆ Drills	❤ 90 min: Long run	Rest or fun active play

	MONDAY Hills, intervals, or fartlek	TUESDAY Recovery	WEDNESDAY Long/aerobic
6	■ 50 min: Fartlek or hill run ◆ Drills and/or strides	♥ 20–30 min: Jog or ✖ 30 min: _____ ● Strength	♥ 40–45 min: Aerobic run ◆ Strides
7	■ 5–6 min intervals X 4 1–2 min walk/jog between intervals Goal: approx. 3 miles at 10K pace ◆ Drills and/or strides	♥ 20–30 min: Jog or ✖ 30 min: _____ ● Strength	♥ 50–55 min: Aerobic run ◆ Strides
8	■ 40–45 min: Fartlek or hill run ◆ Drills and/or strides	♥ 20–30 min: Jog or ✖ 30 min: _____ ● Strength	♥ 60 min: Aerobic run including 3 to 4 mile MAFT ◆ Strides
9	■ 40–45 min: Fartlek or hill run ◆ Drills and/or strides	♥ 20–30 min: Jog or ✖ 30 min: _____ ● Strength	♥ 60 min: Aerobic run ◆ Strides
10	■ 8 min intervals X 3 Goal: approx. 3 miles at 10K pace 1–2 min walk/jog between intervals ◆ Drills and/or strides	♥ 20–30 min: Jog or ✖ 30 min: _____ ● Strength	♥ 70 min: Aerobic run ◆ Strides
11	■ 50–55 min: Fartlek or hill run ◆ Drills and/or Strides	♥ 20–30 min: Jog or ✖ 30 min: _____ ● Strength	♥ 70 min: Aerobic run ◆ Strides

THURSDAY	FRIDAY	SATURDAY	SUNDAY
Recovery	Aerobic	Tempo or long run	Recovery
❤ 20–30 min: Jog or ✖ 30 min: ● Strength	❤ 45 min: Jog ◆ Drills	■ 55 min: Tempo run *Go out easy, finish fast and strong* ◆ Drills and/or strides	Rest or fun active play
❤ 20–30 min: Jog or ✖ 30 min: ● Strength	❤ 50 min: Jog ◆ Drills	❤ 100–120 min: Long run	Rest or fun active play
❤ 20–30 min: Jog or ✖ 30 min: ● Strength	❤ 50 min: Jog ◆ Drills	❤ 60–90 min: Long run	Rest or fun active play
❤ 20–30 min: Jog or ✖ 30 min: ● Strength	❤ 50 min: Jog ◆ Drills	■ 55 min: Tempo run *Go out easy, finish fast and strong* ◆ Drills and/or strides	Rest or fun active play
❤ 20–30 min: Jog or ✖ 30 min: ● Strength	❤ 50–60 min: Jog ◆ Drills	❤ 100–120 min: Long run	Rest or fun active play
❤ 20–30 min: Jog or ✖ 30 min: ● Strength	❤ 50–60 min: Jog ◆ Drills	■ 60 min: Tempo run *Go out easy, finish fast and strong* ◆ Drills and/or strides	Rest or fun active play

	MONDAY	TUESDAY	WEDNESDAY
	Hills, intervals, or fartlek	Recovery	Long/aerobic
12	■ 45–50 min: Fartlek or hill run ◆ Drills and/or Strides	♥ 20–30 min: Jog or ✖ 30 min: ——— ● Strength	♥ 60 min: Aerobic run including 3 to 4 mile MAFT ◆ Strides

13	■ 5–6 min intervals X 4
	  1–2 min walk/jog between intervals
	  Goal: approx. 3 miles at 10K pace
	◆ Drills and/or strides
		♥ 20–30 min: Jog or
		✖ 30 min:
		
		———
		● Strength
			♥ 75 min: Aerobic run
			◆ Strides

14	■ 45–50 min: Fartlek or hill run ◆ Drills and/or strides	♥ 20–30 min: Jog or ✖ 30 min: ——— ● Strength	♥ 70 min: Aerobic run ◆ Strides
15	■ 45–50 min: Fartlek or hill run ◆ Drills and/or strides	♥ 20–30 min: Jog or ✖ 30 min: ——— ● Strength	♥ 45–50 min: Aerobic run including 3 to 4 mile MAFT ◆ Strides

16	■ 4 min intervals X 3
	  2–3 min walk/jog between intervals
	  Stay relaxed, keeping some speed in taper
	◆ Drills and/or strides
		♥ 20–30 min: Jog or
		✖ 30 min:
		
		———
		● Strength
			♥ 30 min: Aerobic run
			◆ Strides

THURSDAY	FRIDAY	SATURDAY	SUNDAY
Recovery	Aerobic	Tempo or long run	Recovery
♥ 20–30 min: Jog or ✖ 30 min: ● Strength	♥ 50–60 min: Jog ◆ Drills	♥ 120 min: Long run	Rest or fun active play
♥ 20–30 min: Jog or ✖ 30 min: ● Strength	♥ 50–60 min: Jog ◆ Drills	■ 55 min: Tempo run *Go out easy, finish fast and strong* ◆ Drills and/or strides	Rest or fun active play
♥ 20–30 min: Jog or ✖ 30 min: ● Strength	♥ 50 min: Jog ◆ Drills	♥ 90 min: Long run	Rest or fun active play
♥ 20–30 min: Jog or ✖ 30 min: ● Strength	♥ 40 min: Jog ◆ Drills	■ 45–50 min: Tempo run *Go out easy, finish fast and strong* ◆ Drills and/or strides	Rest or fun active play
Rest	♥ 30 min: Easy run ◆ Strides	Rest	■ **Marathon Day!**

OVERVIEW OF THE KEY PARTS OF
THE THREE RUNNING PROGRAMS

Aerobic runs

Aerobic runs are the foundation of fitness and health. Run at or slightly below your maximum aerobic heart rate (MAHR) for the duration of the run—a speed at which you should be able to easily converse. At least 80 percent of your running should be done at or below your MAHR—until four to six weeks prior to an event or PT test. The first ten minutes of the aerobic runs in this plan are intended as a relaxed warm-up and to gradually raise your heart rate toward your MAHR. When you finish these runs, you should feel as if you could run more.

To find your maximum aerobic heart rate, use Dr. Phil Maffetone's 180 Formula. Example below is a thirty-year-old runner.

1. Subtract your age from 180 (example: 180 – 30 = 150).
2. Modify this number by selecting the option below that best matches your health profile:
   a. If you have, or are recovering from, a major illness or are taking medication, subtract an additional 10 (example: 150 – 10 = 140).
   b. If you have not exercised before, have been training inconsistently or been injured, have not recently progressed in training or competition, get more than two colds or bouts of flu per year, or have allergies, subtract an additional 5 (example: 140 – 5 = 135).
   c. If you've been exercising regularly (at least four times weekly) for up to two years without any of the problems listed in a. and b., keep the number the same as in 1 (example: 180 – 30 = 150).
   d. If you have been competing for more than two years without any of the problems listed above and have improved in competition without injury, add 5 (example: 180 – 30 + 5 = 155).

Body adaptation: Aerobic development. Growth of capillaries and mitochondria. Increased fat-burning capacity. Relaxed running form.

Common mistakes:
- Ignoring your MAHR and your level of effort. (When you run above your MAHR, you are burning mostly glucose/glycogen, tapping into anaerobic metabolism, and inhibiting aerobic development.)
- Trying to run at a fixed pace.
- Going too fast up hills.

Long runs

Long, slow runs (longer than one hour) are a significant aerobic stimulus. Time on your feet is the goal—not speed. In a sugar-depleted "fasting" state (no carbohydrates before or during the run), you'll teach your body to burn fat and recruit more muscle fibers—that is, you will recruit fast twitch aerobic muscle fibers as slow twitch muscles fatigue. You should take a long run no more than once every one to two weeks.

Start comfortably below your MAHR. On the return leg, you may run at your MAHR. Slowly build up your pace, and slowly extend the time on your feet to an hour and a half (two hours for experienced runners).

Maintain adequate hydration by following your thirst cues—not overdrinking, as this can lead to hyponatremia—a life-threatening condition that occurs when your sodium levels are too low. Replace fluids with a good recovery meal shortly after a long run, preferably within half an hour. As you get closer to race day, if you're feeling good, do the second half of your long runs at near-marathon pace.

Body adaptation: Aerobic development. Growth of capillaries and mitochondria. Increased fat-burning capacity and relaxed running form. Longer runs, even though you may feel comfortable and are not pushing very hard, stimulate maximum muscle recruitment.

Common mistakes:
- Running too fast so that you finish fatigued (and slow). As with all training runs, you should feel as if you could turn around and do this run again if you had to.

- Starting out above your MAHR and tapping out your glucose reserves, instead of stimulating your fat burning capability.
- Relying on carbs for energy, rather than training your body to mobilize fat as fuel.
- Making a single long run more than 50 percent of your weekly miles.

Jog (slow jog)

The jogs in this plan help you recover and focus on a relaxed and efficient movement pattern. They're also good for mental relaxation, stress reduction, and general health. You should run much more slowly than you're capable of, below your MAHR. Use a light, springy running motion, and keep your cadence close to 180 steps per minute. The goal is an easy twenty to thirty minutes of activity.

Body adaptation: Aerobic development and recovery. You are training the movement pattern as you focus on form, breathing, and relaxation. This easy activity stimulates your parasympathetic nervous system, which is essential for moderating stress.

Common mistakes:
- Timing your jog for speed.
- Getting frustrated with the slow pace.
- Running above your MAHR.

Threshold or tempo run

The threshold is the top-end aerobic pace, right at the line between aerobic and anaerobic—the fastest you can run without generating more acidity than you can recycle back into energy. Called the anaerobic threshold, this is the pace you could sustain for at least thirty up to sixty minutes once you are fit (around the pace for a 10K run).

For these runs, warm up nice and easy for at least ten minutes with a relaxed jog.

Choose an out-and-back or loop course you enjoy that is uninterrupted by traffic. A track works well for shorter distances. Run at comfortable, hard effort, building from fifteen minutes up to thirty minutes. Your effort and heart rate (if you wear a heart rate monitor) should be constant from week to week. (As you become more efficient, your pace will increase naturally.)

Body adaptation: Relaxed speed. Improved running economy; improved aerobic development (remember, this is below anaerobic threshold). Improved understanding of pacing.

Common mistakes:
- Running "all out" or thinking of it as a race.
- Checking your watch and wanting to follow specific times.
- Thinking you need to improve time with each successive run. Instead, think *fast and relaxed.*

Fartlek

Running should be fun. A fartlek is a type of fun running that was first done in Sweden in the 1930s and is practiced by runners and coaches to this day. The word literally means "speed play."

Speed up and slow down according to how you feel—not by any set pace or time interval. This is how a child runs. Make the recovery portions relaxed. This is a great way to work on form, relaxation, dynamic stretching, and strength.

Make it up as you go. Run quick and relaxed to telephone poles, up hills, to a target that you randomly pick out. Like play, there is no time or distance outcome. The fast segments can be thirty seconds to a few minutes, with the total run time between twenty and forty minutes, or longer once you're fit and ready. Pick a fun, scenic route with little traffic. Warm up for ten minutes, then run the whole mix of paces over an undulating terrain. Mix in some sprints, hills, and strides for a minute or two, then recover between the speed segments. Keep your level of effort below the anaerobic threshold. Cool down for ten minutes.

Body adaptation: Aerobic development and coordination. Relaxed leg speed. Increasing strength (especially if you include sprinting up some hills).

Common mistakes:
- Making this a structured workout with a set time or pace.
- Making this hard and anaerobic for long segments.
- Not recovering between speed segments.

Intervals

Intervals improve your ability to run at your anaerobic threshold and teach you to buffer acidity (which is easier because of your already-large aerobic base). They also help you rehearse race speeds, without being overly taxing. The goal is to feel that you have made a strong effort, but haven't gone all out.

To run intervals, start by warming up for ten minutes with a jog and then some light, quick, short strides. Then choose a distance or duration—measured in minutes or laps—for a higher level of effort that you feel comfortable repeating (with a recovery period after each). The total time of faster running intervals (broken into segments) can be five minutes for the beginner, and up to twenty minutes for the more advanced runner. The recovery (slower running) period should be of equal time to the faster interval. (When doing intervals for long-distance training, however, the recovery rest time can be shorter than your interval.) Allow your heart rate to recover to 120–130 bpm—until you feel ready to go again. Stop the workout if you struggle to hold your pace or suspect that your form is compromised.

You should always end this workout feeling as if you could do another interval if you had to. Cool down with an easy ten-minute jog.

Body adaptation: Relaxed speed. Good pacing. Elevated anaerobic threshold, and tolerance to oxygen debt.

Common mistakes:
- Trying to run a set time, and running all out and too fast. Times are not important. You're working for physiological and strength adaptations.
- Too short of a recovery jog.
- Trying to race (or keep up with) a group above your level.

Hills

Many runners fear hills and avoid them. But running up and down hills at a comfortable pace, with good technique, develops strength. It's like a free gym workout—outside! And running downhill is a fun way to develop relaxed speed and work on form.

The course can be a loop with a couple of hills ranging from a hundred meters to a half mile. If you're lucky to live in the mountains, you can climb for a couple of miles and then run swiftly down. As a beginner, don't try to run fast on the uphills. Remain tall with your chest up and open. Look forward, but resist the tendency to look down and bend at the waist. Keep your stride short, and use your glutes to push and spring off the ground.

Practice running efficiently and quickly on the downhills. Think: *Run over the ground and not into the ground.* On the uphills, your heart rate will exceed your MAHR, but should remain below your anaerobic threshold.

Body adaptation: Leg strength (uphill); leg speed, coordination, and mobility (downhill). Aerobic development.

Common mistakes:
- Running too fast and straining on the hills—at the expense of good form and going into oxygen debt.
- Running too hard (with high impact) on the downhills. Remember: good downhill running is a skill.

Strides

Strides, also known as pickups, develop speed and coordination. This is a form of dynamic stretching, coordination, and strength work over short distances. No acidity accumulates. It should be fun! All animals (humans included) love short sprints. Strides make you a better runner for both short and long events.

After a thorough warm-up, during a run, or at the end of a run, do four to eight pickups of 50 to 80 meters by gradually speeding up to a sprint, then slowing back down. A grass field is ideal. Accelerate naturally and progressively, and decelerate slowly. Give yourself a full recovery between each pickup, even though these aren't a true workout. The goal is to not develop acidity or fatigue. Each sprint should feel progressively easier and quicker as you loosen up. Focus on form and relaxed speed.

Body adaptation: Strengthens and adds mobility to the key running muscles and tendons. Develops coordination and skill.

Common mistakes:
- Running too hard and long during the strides, such that your form breaks down.
- Not recovering between strides (and allowing acidity to build in muscles).
- Thinking of these as "workouts" that need to be done harder and faster each time.
- Attempting high-intensity interval training (HIIT) before you feel coordinated, strong, pain-free, and safe in your strides. The reward of HIIT is high, but so is the risk if your form and function are not correct.

Drills

The drills in this program first develop coordination through repetition of correct movement. As you progress, they add strength and mobility. As with sprints, these should be fun and a bit challenging!

Work on mastering the movement before trying to add speed or power to the drills. A grass field is the ideal surface. Give yourself a full recovery between sets. Beginning runners following the 5K plan should stick with jumping rope, lateral jumps, four square, heel lifts, grapevines, and razor scooter (for correct form, review the videos at runforyourlifebook.com). If you have access to a TrueForm Runner, spend some time on it!

Those following our half-marathon and marathon plans can progress to tougher drills, such as ABCD skips, running in place with a tether, and more. Execute your drills a few times a week, or even daily at the end of a run. Mix it up. Have fun.

Body adaptation: Strengthens and adds mobility to the key muscles and tendons used in running. Develops running skills and coordination.

Common mistakes:
- Doing drills with incorrect form.
- Not recovering between sets.
- Applying power before mastering the movement.

Cross-train

Pick a time to dedicate thirty minutes to a relaxed, enjoyable activity. Swimming, biking, CrossFit, gym work, yoga, hiking . . . it's all good as long as it's not stressful, and it promotes relaxation and recovery.

The American College of Sports Medicine recommends that everyone try to get thirty minutes of physical activity daily with the safe guideline of increasing running volume no more than 10 percent a week. Different activities allow you to recover from the tissue stresses of running, especially for the beginner. Cross-training isn't specific to running, though, so don't assume that it will greatly assist you in passing your PT test.

Body adaptation: Continued aerobic development, as well as sport-specific strength.

Common mistakes:
- Going too hard on recovery cross-training days.
- Using poor technique in the cross-training activity, adding to existing mechanical stress on tissues.
- Assuming that the cross-training will make you run faster.
- If you are using cross-training during an injury, assuming that when the injury is healed you can jump back into the same volume and intensity of running as you were doing in cross-training sessions. The tissue load of running is different, even if you are "fit."

Pre-event practice race
This is a race simulation done at a comfortably hard running pace, but not all out. The goal is to develop rhythm, relaxation, and pacing at higher speeds, while maximally tapping your aerobic system. (You may become slightly anaerobic, which helps develop tolerance to acidity and fatigue.) This can be done at an actual race too. A half marathon is a good practice race for a marathon.

This should be done four to six weeks out from your event, and you can make it one of your long runs around that time. It will build confidence in what you can do on the day of your event. In fact, try to replicate what you will do on race day. Wear similar clothes and footwear, find a similar course, eat similarly, and warm up for ten minutes. Do a few light strides. Do not stretch. Try using positive affirmations before and during the run. Chart your progress!

Body adaptation: An elevated anaerobic threshold, and rehearsal for relaxed speed.

Common mistakes:
- Going 100 percent. Try 95 percent. Finish strong and save your best for event day.
- Starting out too fast, then slowing at the end.
- Trying to run faster each time.

Maximum aerobic function test (MAFT)

(Used with permission of Dr. Phil Maffetone.)

This test measures improvements in aerobic speed (at the same time that you are working on building your foundation for aerobic running). If you are running faster at the same aerobic heart rate, it means you are building aerobic speed. Without an objective measurement, you can fool yourself into thinking you're progressing.

Perform the MAFT on a track or measured flat distance with your heart rate monitor, by running at the maximum aerobic heart rate (MAHR) found with Dr. Maffetone's 180 Formula. A distance of three to five miles will provide good data, although a one-mile test still has value. Do the test following an easy warm-up.

Below is an example of a baseline MAFT performed by running on a track, at a constant heart rate of 145, in minutes per mile:

Mile 1: 11:32
Mile 2: 11:46
Mile 3: 11:49

Beginning runners should do a MAFT regularly. Others should perform the test now and then throughout the year. For instance:

	Baseline	September	October	November
Mile 1:	11:32	10:29	9:35	9:10
Mile 2:	11:46	10:46	9:43	9:22
Mile 3:	11:49	10:44	9:47	9:31

Chart your progress, and note the improvement!

Body adaptation: Growth of capillaries, mitochondria, fat-burning capacity, and more relaxed running form. Your aerobic system is improving, enabling you to run faster with the same effort. Your times will slowly improve!

Common mistakes:
- Running different courses in different conditions for the test. For instance, a hot, windy day won't result in the same time (at the same effort) as a cool, calm day.
- Doing the test on a day when you're fatigued.
- Not warming up.
- Choosing too long of a distance when you are first starting this test. One or two miles is good for a new runner.
- "Cheating" and running faster than your predetermined MAHR.

Appendix IV

A SELECTION OF BOOKS ON RUNNING AND HEALTHY LIVING

Here are some of what I've found to be the best reads on the art and science of exercise physiology, running mechanics, footwear, injury prevention, and training for runners of all ages and abilities.

The Big Book of Endurance Training and Racing and *The Big Book of Health and Fitness,* by Dr. Philip Maffetone. These two books are must-reads for understanding the basics of aerobic versus anaerobic activity, as well as ADS (aerobic deficiency syndrome). Maffetone trained legendary athletes Mark Allen, Mike Pigg, and Stu Mittleman. The principles that he outlines—including important sections on diet—work equally well for entry-level and high-level runners.

Anatomy for Runners, by Jay Dicharry. This is *the* tool kit for runners, coaches, and the medical providers who are treating them. Learn how your body works, and how to reset it to achieve better health. (Jay has worked closely with me on the USAF Efficient Running project.)

Tread Lightly, by Peter Larson and Bill Katovsky. This book nicely covers the science of running and running shoes, as well as the scientific principles of running form, the effects of footwear, and healthier running in general. Our work here is highlighted throughout this book.

Your Best Stride and *Run Strong, Stay Hungry,* by Jonathan Beverly. A good friend for many years and former editor of *Running Times* shares simple lessons from many of the best runners over the past fifty years. I'm proud to have a part in both of these books.

Healthy Intelligent Training, by Keith Livingstone. The time-tested Lydiard Method is outlined in this insightful volume, with easy-to-follow instructions. These are the lessons and methods of the Coach of Champions, who helped introduce "jogging" to America.

The Oxygen Advantage, by Patrick McKeown. This book got me thinking about the effects of optimal versus poor breathing not just for sports and my own life, but for the care of my medical patients. Not a day goes by when I'm not sharing something from this book. We all need to breathe.

Whole Body Barefoot, Simple Steps to Foot Pain Relief, Movement Matters, and *Move Your DNA,* by Katy Bowman. This prolific writer and movement specialist carefully shows how our modern lifestyle is killing us. These four books are a good primer on the importance of the feet, how to move more of *them,* and more of *you.*

Primal Endurance, by Mark Sisson and Brad Kearns. Ancestral principles applied to food, movement, sleep, stress, and longevity. Become a fat-burning beast!

Slow Jogging, by Hiroaki Tanaka. I had the privilege of writing the foreword to this important and insightful book about the value of slow jogging as the path back to health and reduction of injuries.

ChiRunning, 2nd edition, by Danny Dreyer. I'm likewise honored to have written the foreword. Danny and I share a passion for learning and understanding the basics of movement.

Challenging Beliefs, by Tim Noakes. A world leader in exercise science challenges much of conventional wisdom on topics of nutrition, hydration, and endurance performance.

Explosive Running, 2nd edition, by Michael Yessis. A clear explanation of how to be fast and efficient.

The Story of the Human Body, by Daniel E. Lieberman. The Harvard evolutionary biologist (and friend), known as the "barefoot professor," explains what our bodies were designed for, focusing on the prevalence of "mismatch diseases" caused by environmental and cultural vectors that we're not adapted for.

Aerobics, by Kenneth H. Cooper. This groundbreaking short book on the science of aerobic health is just as relevant today as when it was released in 1968.

Jogging, by William J. Bowerman and W. E. Harris. Legendary New Zealand coach Arthur Lydiard inspired Bill Bowerman, a cofounder of Nike, to introduce jogging to America. Soon thousands were running for fun and health. Go forward by looking back!

Serious Runner's Handbook, by Tom Osler. A slim, commonsense guide to healthy running, published in 1976, that is still relevant today.

Human Locomotion and *Injury-Free Running,* by Thomas C. Michaud. Epic reads for anyone treating runners in a health care setting, by the illustrator for this book.

8 Steps to a Pain-Free Back, by Esther Gokhale. Relearn how to sit, stand, and walk.

Running and Being, by Dr. George Sheehan. A classic work by the original doctor/runner/philosopher/exercise authority.

Long Distance, by Bill McKibben. A great read on the principles of exercise physiology and the mind to endure.

Why We Run, by Bernd Heinrich. For the anthropologist in us all. How can birds fly for thousands of miles on minimal food? By burning efficient and tasty fat.

Lore of Running, by Dr. Tim Noakes. Explains the science of running in detail. The fourth edition is considered the bible of running.

Born to Run and *Natural Born Heroes,* by Christopher McDougall. The *New York Times* bestselling author tells the tale of an injured runner discovering the secrets of the legendary Tarahumara of Mexico and the secrets of the legendary citizen soldiers of Crete.

Spark: The Revolutionary New Science of Exercise and the Brain, by John Ratey. A groundbreaking and fascinating investigation of the transformative effects of exercise on the brain.

Play: How It Shapes the Brain, Opens the Imagination, and Invigorates the Soul, by Stuart Brown. An excellent book on the science of play and its essential role in a life of happiness and intelligence.

Anatomy Trains: Myofascial Meridians for Manual and Movement Therapists, by Thomas Myers. This book will change the way you view the human body and how it moves. We all need to understand how to maintain our fascia, the vital web that integrates our body's communication with its movement.

Fit Soul, Fit Body, by Brandt Segunda and Mark Allen. A six-time Ironman winner reflects on the essentials of sustainable activity and health. Discover the connection between mind, body, and soul.

The Nature Fix, by Florence Williams. Without vitamin "N," it is rare for any positive health change to occur. An in-depth dive into the science of the outdoors, suitable for reading in the sunshine or in the shade of a tree.

And a few of my favorites on diet and nutrition:

The Overfat Pandemic, by Dr. Philip Maffetone. Emerging research shows that the overfat pandemic is alarmingly prevalent in developed countries, where up to 80 percent of adults and 50 percent of children suffer from this condition.

Fat Chance: Beating the Odds Against Sugar, Processed Food, Obesity, and Disease, by Robert Lustig, M.D. An excellent overview and disquisition for anyone who wants to understand the science of food and obesity. This is required reading for our medical students.

Why We Get Fat and What to Do About It; Good Calories, Bad Calories; and *The Case Against Sugar,* by Gary Taubes. Three eye-opening, myth-shattering examinations of what makes us fat, from the acclaimed science writer.

Deep Nutrition, by Catherine Shanahan, M.D. Affectionately known as "Dr. Cate" to the Los Angeles Lakers and other professional sports teams, she was an innovator who connected healthy food to human performance in a transformative way, for those whose careers depend on it.

In Defense of Food and *Food Rules,* by Michael Pollan. This eloquent manifesto and follow-up handbook show how we can start making thoughtful food choices that will enrich our lives, enlarge our sense of what it means to be healthy, and bring pleasure back to eating.

Nutrition and Physical Degeneration, by Weston A. Price. A classic work from the 1930s on nutrition and its effects on health, based on Price's studies of the healthiest places on earth.

Always Hungry?, by David Ludwig, M.D. From one of the world's leading obesity clinicians and researchers. Overeating does not make you fat.

The Big Fat Surprise, by Nina Teicholz. Nina challenges the establishment. Ten years of work went into this impeccably researched challenge to those who suggest that dietary fat is the cause of obesity and disease.

Eat Fat, Get Thin, by Mark Hyman, M.D., of the Cleveland Clinic. More simple truth about what is wrong with nutrition science, and a simple way to start in a new direction.

Wired to Eat and *The Paleo Solution,* by Robb Wolf. Robb works with me to help Native Americans and first responders, and he dives into the science and ancestral health principles of food, and of how we live in the modern world.

The Art and Science of Low Carbohydrate Living and *The Art and Science of Low Carbohydrate Performance,* by Drs. Stephen Phinney and Jeff Volek. These two books are *the* scientific and practical references for a low-carb diet.

The Real Meal Revolution, vols. 1 and 2, by Tim Noakes and Jonno Proudfoot. Dr. Noakes is changing the world from South Africa, where "Banting" is becoming an everyday term for a healthy, low-carb way of eating.

The New Atkins for a New You, by Drs. Eric Westman, Stephen Phinney, and Jeff Volek. This book lends more science and refinement to the original Atkins Diet, by three of the top clinicians and researchers in the fields of obesity and metabolism.

Diabetes Unpacked, by Zoe Harcombe, Ph.D., and

colleagues. The world's leading researchers on diabetes and metabolism make the case for changing the government nutrition guidelines that are driving this chronic disease.

And for kids and youth:

The Youth and Teen Running Encyclopedia, by Mick Grant. This disciple of Arthur Lydiard presents the philosophy of fun first—so that kids want to come back to practice and never get hurt running.

Super Food for Superchildren, by Dr. Tim Noakes, Jonno Proudfoot, and Bridget Surtees. With childhood obesity at epidemic levels and no reversal of the trend in sight, we need to make food healthy and fun again, and teach families to cook meals that are free of added sugar and processed carbs.

Fat Head Kids, by Tom Naughton. Based on the humorous but startlingly real documentary *Fat Head,* this book demonstrates that much of the official advice about healthy eating is wrong, and has created a record number of overweight youth who can't concentrate in school. This book makes getting healthy fun.

Just Let the Kids Play, by Bob Bigelow. A must-read for parents, this book singles out our elite focused youth sports programs as the cause of the problem, and offers practical ways to rebuild them so they better serve the physical and emotional needs of children.

Appendix V

THE TEN ESSENTIAL ELEMENTS OF HEALTHY RUNNING

IMAGINE MOVING PAIN-FREE FOR A LIFETIME. IT'S EASY IF YOU TRY.

1. Preassess yourself
If you have cardiac risk, a medical condition, are taking medications, or are injured, speak to a health professional you trust before you embark on or escalate physical activity.

2. Follow the general principles of natural and healthy running
Train the endurance engine, have fun, move your whole body, sprint a little, progress gradually, go barefoot or minimal with your footwear, and eat real food. Set the intention of doing that— often—for the rest of your life!

3. Give yourself positive affirmations
Activate the power of the mind through repetition of positive statements. (You can use "I" or "you." I prefer "you.") Create your own affirmations—those are the best—and repeat them daily. For example: *You are powerful and springy. You love the hills.*

4. Warm up
Give yourself ten minutes to warm up, at an easy, comfortable pace. Become springy and bouncy and loose. Listen to your body—it will tell you when you are ready.

5. Keep the movement going
Develop your personal daily mobility routine, and keep doing it. Mine takes five minutes every morning—the perfect launch pad for an energetic, productive day.

6. Prevent injury

Be aware of a tendency to build endurance prior to gaining structural strength in muscles, ligaments, bones, and tendons. The body will adapt to stresses, as long as the load is not greater than its capacity to adapt. So include strength and mobility in your endurance building.

7. Recover

Balancing stress and allowing time for recovery is essential. Running should fit into the relaxing part of the day, not add to daily stress.

8. Monitor the signs of improving fitness and health

How are you feeling, and what do the simple measurements say? If your waistline, blood glucose level, and blood pressure are improving, and your level of vigor, too—you're on the right track. And try a heart rate monitor—a form of biofeedback that helps in listening to your body. Learn the language of your physiology.

9. You can't outrun a bad diet

Avoid eating crap. Junk food and excess sugar will sabotage every effort to become and remain healthy and stay young. Just say no to sweetened drinks.

10. Set a goal

Where are you now? Where do you want to be? *Why* have you set this goal? Once you achieve your short-term goals with comfort and confidence, work toward sustainable, longer-term goals.

Acknowledgments

This book represents the distilled essence of an adult lifetime—not merely of running but of exploring the function and physiology of the human body. Such a task couldn't have been undertaken alone. I am indebted to my running and medical colleagues not only for sharing valuable knowledge and experience for this book, but for their guidance and friendship throughout my career: in particular, Dr. Ray McClanahan, who taught me about the foot, and Dr. Daniel Lieberman, the premier authority on evolutionary biology and health.

For helping me find my stride, and for sharing what we do with so many, I'd like to thank running education colleagues Ian Adamson, Jay Dicharry, Blaise Dubois, Dr. Lawrence van Lingen, Dr. Irene Davis, Dr. Trent Nessler, Dr. Ken Mierke, Lorraine Moller, Rod Dixon, Nobby Hashizume (Lydiard Foundation), Danny Dreyer, Chris McDougall, Lee Saxby, and Danny Abshire. To my nutrition colleagues Dr. Tim Noakes, Nina Teicholz, Gary Taubes, Dr. Eric Westman, Dr. Robert Lustig, Dr. Joseph Scherger, Dr. Robert Oh, Dr. Sarah Hallberg, Dr. Cate Shanahan, Dr. Stephen Phinney, Dr. Jeff Volek, Sami Inkinin, Dr. Jeff Gerber, Jimmy Moore—and many others who are now teaching and sharing the knowledge that patients can reverse metabolic illness. And, to West Virginia University colleagues Dr. KC Nau, Dr. Emma Eggleston, Dr. Clay Marsh, and Dr. Rosemarie Lorenzetti: thank you for your commitment to promoting food as medicine.

I'd especially like to thank running colleagues Jonathan Beverly, Brian Metzler, Amby Burfoot, Dr. Peter Snell, Keith Livingston, Roberto Ruiz, Chris Fall, Curt Munson, George Banker, Dave McGillivray, Dr. Nick Campitelli, Don Freeman, Scott Warr, Golden Harper, Dr. Casey Kerrigan, Tony Post, Steve Sashen, Sara Davidson, Kimberly Bachmeier, Elinor Fish, Sarah Young, Mick Grant, and Jerry Lee for your research, teaching, writing, podcasts, and innovation in the running realm.

In particular, I'd like to thank the late Bill Katovsky and Nicholas Pang for helping me create the Natural Running Center, and Jeff Vernon and Robin Desjardins for creating TrueForm runner training, which makes learning to run easier.

I'd also like to thank my local community, who have faithfully supported our mission at Two Rivers Treads and Freedom's Run, and contributed stories and anecdotes for this book: Lois Turco, Holly Fry, Dr. Andro Barnett, Dr. Stacey Kendig, Katie Nolan Thompson, Morgan Wright, Candus Sutphin, Sarah Hodder, Diana Gorham, Dion Navarra, Erin Gaertner, Paul Koczera, Bill Susa, Jeff and Sheri Fiolek, Katherine Cobb, Kevin and Jennie Brakens, Susan Reichel, Bill Bondurant, James and Suzy Munnis, Jared Matlick, Fiona Harrison, James Hersick, Antonio Eppolito, Paul Encarnacion, Pat Schneble, Matt Knott, Mick Brown, Laura Bergman, Pat Fore, and Lara Foster.

Special thanks go to key contributors to this book, who have also been lifetime mentors to me and many others: Dr. Phil Maffetone, an internationally recognized coach and healer, and Dr. Tom Michaud—master of anatomy, clinician, inventor, and author. I am also proud to feature the professional photographic work of Joel Wolpert, a fellow West Virginian.

The critical partner in this book project was my writing collaborator, Broughton Coburn. Brot in turn would like to thank Dr. Tom Barrett and Dr. Polly Fabian, for their careful and informative technical review; Mari Siceloff for sharing her experience in coaching and running marathons; Susan Koskinen for library research; and his wife, Didi Thunder; daughter, Phoebe Coburn; and son, Tenzing Coburn, for their research assistance.

Finally, this could not have been done without the support of my family. My wife, Roberta, and children, Leo and Lily, have tolerated, with friendly humor, my barefoot-running and low-carb lifestyle, and the hours of work required to grow and shape this book. And unending thanks to my parents, Vincent and Nancy Cucuzzella, who gave my brothers and me the opportunity to go outside to run and play.

Notes

Inttroduction

xviii How can we become healthier: With many thanks to my physical therapy colleague Jay Dicharry, author of *Anatomy for Runners,* who developed this construct.

CHAPTER 1 Our Bodies Are Older Than We Think

3 12,000 years as pastoralists and farmers: See the Genographic Project of the National Geographic Society: https://genographic.nationalgeographic.com/.

5 evolutionary adaptations in our anatomy: See, for instance, Dennis Bramble and Daniel Lieberman, "Endurance Running and the Evolution of *Homo,*" *Nature* 432, no. 7015 (2004): 345–52, and Daniel Lieberman et al., "Foot Strike Patterns and Collision Forces in Habitually Barefoot versus Shod Runners," *Nature* 463, no. 7280 (2010): 531–36.

10 Despite all this medical attention: See "Life Expectancy Climbs Worldwide but People Spend More Years Living with Illness and Disability," news release, Institute for Health Metrics and Evaluation, University of Washington, Seattle, 2013. Also GBD 2015 DALYs and HALE Collaborators, "Global, Regional, and National Disability-Adjusted Life-Years (DALYs) for 315 Diseases and Injuries and Healthy Life Expectancy (HALE), 1990–2015: A Systematic Analysis for the Global Burden of Disease Study 2015," *Lancet* 388, no. 10053 (2016): 1603–58.

CHAPTER 2 Stand Up and Breathe

20 elevating the risk of metabolic diseases: Marc T. Hamilton, Deborah G. Hamilton, and Theodore W. Zderic, "Exercise Physiology versus Inactivity Physiology: An Essential Concept for Understanding Lipoprotein Lipase Regulation," *Exercise and Sport Sciences Reviews* 32, no. 4 (2004): 161–66.

CHAPTER 8 Move More and "Exercise" Less

117 Emerging research that traces the roles: From T. W. Zderic and M. T. Hamilton, "Identification of Hemostatic Genes Expressed in Human and Rat Leg Muscles and a Novel Gene (LPP1/PAP2A) Suppressed During Prolonged Physical Inactivity (Sitting)," *Lipids in Health and Disease* 11, no. 137 (2015). "Physical inactivity is an established risk factor for some blood clotting disorders. The effects of inactivity during sitting are most alarming when a person develops the enigmatic condition in the legs called deep venous thrombosis (DVT) or 'couch syndrome,' caused in part by muscular inactivity . . . These findings suggest that skeletal muscle may play an important role in hemostasis and that muscular inactivity may contribute to hemostatic disorders not only because of the slowing of blood flow per se, but also potentially because of the contribution from genes expressed locally in muscles, such as LPP1."

118   At home, I rarely sit in chairs: See Steve Chandler's demonstration, "Sit Better to Move Better," at breakingmuscle.com/fitness.

118   Gene expression, we're learning: The PMC, or primary motor cortex, is where conscious thoughts are translated into movement. The central pattern generator (CPG), in the central cortex, controls "automatic," reflexive actions. After three thousand to thirty thousand repetitions, a consciously controlled movement gets woven into the CPG. See K. Minassian et al., "The Human Central Pattern Generator for Locomotion," *Neuroscientist* 23, no. 6 (2017): 649–63.

CHAPTER 9 Eating to Go the Distance

141   Essentially, fructose metabolism: Sam Z. Sun and Mark W. Empie, "Fructose Metabolism in Humans—What Isotopic Tracer Studies Tell Us," *Nutrition & Metabolism* 9, no. 89 (2012). "Glucose utilization can be regulated before cleavage, whereas fructose is less regulated. This initial difference has prompted some to hypothesize that, because fructose cleavage bypasses key feedback regulatory steps in the glucose metabolic pathway, this bypass may lead to increases of fatty acid synthesis, which may contribute to causes of obesity. This hypothesis relies on a simplified metabolic pathway analysis and on studies using pure fructose in comparison to pure glucose, a situation which rarely occurs in the American diet." With thanks to Cate Shanahan for reviewing this section.

143   the prevalence of diabetes: S. Basu et al., "The Relationship of Sugar to Population-Level Diabetes Prevalence: An Econometric Analysis of Repeated Cross-Sectional Data," *PLoS ONE* 8, no. 2 (2013).

144   The most likely suspect: James J. DiNicolantonio, Sean C. Lucan, and James H. O'Keefe, "The Evidence for Saturated Fat and for Sugar Related to Coronary Heart Disease," *Progress in Cardiovascular Diseases* 58, no. 5 (2016): 464–72.

144   The recent PURE (Prospective Urban Rural Epidemiology) study: Mahshid Dehghan et al., "Association of Fats and Carbohydrate Intake with Cardiovascular Disease and Mortality in 18 Countries from Five Continents (PURE): A Prospective Cohort Study," *The Lancet* 390, no. 10107 (2017): 2050–62.

145   Now each of us consumes over 125 pounds of sugar: James J. DiNicolantonio and Amy Berger, "Added Sugars Drive Nutrient and Energy Deficit in Obesity: A New Paradigm," *Open Heart* 3 (2016).

146   a high fructose load on the liver: Gianluca Perseghin, "Viewpoints on the Way to a Consensus Session: Where Does Insulin Resistance Start? The Liver," *Diabetes Care* 32, no. 2 (2009): S164–S167.

146   Dr. Robert Lustig recently published a study: Robert H. Lustig et al., "Isocaloric Fructose Restriction and Metabolic Improvement in Children with Obesity and Metabolic Syndrome," *Obesity* 24 (2016): 453–60.

150   Sodium is prevalent in our diets: James J. DiNicolantonio and Sean C. Lucan, "The Wrong White Crystals: Not Salt but Sugar as Aetiological in Hypertension and Cardiometabolic Disease," *Open Heart* 1 (2014). "One fact about which there is little debate is that the predominant sources of sodium in the diet are industrially processed foods. Processed foods also happen to be generally high in added sugars, the consumption of which might be more strongly and directly associated with hypertension and cardiometabolic risk. Evidence from epidemiological studies and experimental trials in animals and humans

suggests that added sugars, particularly fructose, may increase blood pressure and blood pressure variability, increase heart rate and myocardial oxygen demand, and contribute to inflammation, insulin resistance and broader metabolic dysfunction."

153 It is this even-chain fat: James J. DiNicolantonio, Ashwin M. Subramonian, and James H. O'Keefe, "Added Fructose as a Principal Driver of Non-Alcoholic Fatty Liver Disease: A Public Health Crisis," *Open Heart* 4, no. 2 (2017).

CHAPTER 10 What's for Dinner

159 "Almost every single nutrient": Quoted in Peter Whoriskey, "The U.S. Government Is Poised to Withdraw Longstanding Warnings About Cholesterol," *Washington Post,* February 10, 2015.

161 dual mandates to advise the public: See Marion Nestle, "Food Lobbies, the Food Pyramid, and U.S. Nutrition Policy," *International Journal of Health Services* 23, no. 3 (1993): 483–96.

161 When we turned from hunting: See Yuval N. Harari, *Sapiens: A Brief History of Humankind* (New York: Harper, 2015).

162 A study led by Christopher Ramsden: Christopher E. Ramsden et al., "Re-evaluation of the Traditional Diet-Heart Hypothesis: Analysis of Recovered Data from Minnesota Coronary Experiment (1968–73)," *BMJ* 353 (2016). "[A]lthough the story of the traditional diet-heart hypothesis did not unfold as predicted, the foods that we eat likely play critical roles in the pathogenesis of many diseases. Given the complexity of biological systems and limitations of our research methods, however, current understanding of the biochemical and clinical effects of foods is rudimentary. The history of the traditional diet-heart hypothesis suggests that nutrition research could be improved by not overemphasizing intermediate biomarkers; cautious interpretation of non-randomized studies; and ensuring timely and complete publication of all randomized controlled trials. Given the limitations of current evidence, the best approach might be one of humility, highlighting limitations of current knowledge and setting a high bar for advising intakes beyond what can be provided by natural diets."

166 an adult obesity rate of close to 40 percent: "State of Obesity Health Report," Trust for America's Health and Robert Wood Johnson Foundation, 2016.

CHAPTER 11 Recovery *Is* the Training

173 too much endurance racing: A. La Gerche, D. J. Rakhit, and G. Claessen, "Exercise and the Right Ventricle: A Potential Achilles' Heel," *Cardiovascular Research* 113, no. 12 (2017): 1499–1508.

177 total sodium per day: James J. DiNicolantonio et al., "Is Salt a Culprit or an Innocent Bystander in Hypertension? A Hypothesis Challenging the Ancient Paradigm," *American Journal of Medicine* 130 (2017): 893–99.

CHAPTER 12 Running a Marathon

197 A note on racing in the heat: If it is going to be hot, you might refer to the piece on "Running in the Heat" at the Natural Running Center (naturalrunningcenter.com) website and published in the *Journal of the American Medical Athletic Association,* which I wrote after the steamy 2012 Boston

Marathon. Also, the home page of the American Medical Athletic Association (AMAA, amaasportsmed.org/) has a link in the lower right on current hydration guidelines.

CHAPTER 13 The Runner's High

204 brain-derived neurotrophic factor: Sama F. Sleiman et al., "Exercise Promotes the Expression of Brain Derived Neurotrophic Factor (BDNF) Through the Action of the Ketone Body β-Hydroxybutyrate," *eLife* 5 (2016).

205 "learned nonuse": Norman Doidge, "Brain, Heal Thyself," *Wall Street Journal,* February 6, 2015.

206 The microbiology isn't well understood: See, for instance, Martin Blaser M.D.'s *Missing Microbes: How the Overuse of Antibiotics Is Fueling Our Modern Plagues* (New York: Henry Holt, 2014) and neurologist David Perlmutter M.D.'s *Brain Maker: The Power of Gut Microbes to Heal and Protect Your Brain—for Life* (New York: Little, Brown, 2015).

206 Everyone wants to avoid stress: See the article links in University of Florida, "Why Stress Might Make It Harder to Lose Fat," *Epoch Times,* January 13, 2016. "Mouse models experiencing metabolic stress produced significantly more betatrophin, and their normal fat-burning processes slowed down markedly. Such observations are significant because they shed new light on the biological mechanisms linking stress, betatrophin, and fat metabolism . . . The results provide experimental evidence that stress makes it harder to break down body fat."

207 Studies with negative or questionable results: Erick H. Turner et al., "Selective Publication of Antidepressant Trials and Its Influence on Apparent Efficacy," *New England Journal of Medicine* 358 (2008): 252–60.

207 beneficial neurotransmitter delivery system: Michael Babyak et al., "Exercise Treatment for Major Depression: Maintenance of Therapeutic Benefit at 10 Months," *Psychosomatic Medicine* 62, no. 5 (2000): 633–38. Also Krista A. Barbour and James A. Blumenthal, "Exercise Training and Depression in Older Adults." *Neurobiology of Aging* 26, no. 1 (2005): 119–23; and Krista A. Barbour, Teresa M. Edenfield, and James A. Blumenthal, "Exercise as a Treatment for Depression and Other Psychiatric Disorders: A Review," *Journal of Cardiopulmonary Rehabilitation and Prevention* 27, no. 6 (2007): 359–67.

207 A crowdsourced hub: See "23 Surprisingly Effective Treatments for Depression (One Year Later)," CureTogether.com, May 3, 2011, https://curetogether .com/blog/2011/05/03/23-surprisingly-effective-treatments-for-depression- one-year-later/.

CHAPTER 14 Outsmart Injuries with Prevention

213 More than half of all runners: See Dick Travisano, "What You Don't Know About Common Sport Injuries Can Really Hurt You," The Sports Injury Doctor, http://www.sportsinjurybulletin.com/archive/0123a-sport-injuries.htm.

213 8.3 million days of missed duty: See N. S. Nye et al., "Description and Rate of Musculoskeletal Injuries in Air Force Basic Military Trainees, 2012–2014," *Journal of Athletic Training* 51, no. 11 (2016): 858–65. Also "Cost of Injuries to the Military," from *Army Medical Surveillance Activity, 2005.*

218 Problem knees account: R. N. Van Gent et al., "Incidence and Determinants

of Lower Extremity Running Injuries in Long Distance Runners: A Systematic Review," *British Journal of Sports Medicine* 41, no. 8 (2007): 469–80.

222 *weaken* the foot: To begin the process of treating fallen arches, I have found a brand called Barefoot Science to be helpful. It has pods centered under the arch to help progressively strengthen the intrinsic foot muscles. Textured insoles are also a promising tool that aids in proprioception.

CHAPTER 15 Women Are Pulling Away from the Pack

236 can readily adapt to burn fat: See Meaghan Brown, "The Longer the Race, the Stronger We Get," *Outside,* May 2017.

237 an emerging, broader term: Margo Mountjoy et al., "The IOC Consensus Statement: Beyond the Female Athlete Triad—Relative Energy Deficiency in Sport (RED-S)," *British Journal of Sports Medicine* 48 (2014): 491–97.

238 Overloading causes more breakdown: See, for instance, W. M. Kohrt et al., "American College of Sports Medicine Position Stand: Physical Activity and Bone Health," *Medicine and Science in Sports and Exercise* 36, no. 11 (2004): 1985–96.

238 Yet a study of women college athletes: Diego Villacis et al., "Prevalence of Abnormal Vitamin D Levels Among Division I NCAA Athletes," *Sports Health* 6, no. 4 (2014): 340–47.

241 a third of U.S. babies: See the CDC's National Center for Health Statistics, "Births—Method of Delivery," 2015, www.cdc.gov/nchs/fastats/.

242 evaluate your HRT options carefully: "Menopausal Hormone Therapy Information," National Institutes of Health, www.nih.gov/health-information/menopausal-hormone-therapy-information.

242 risks of running during menopause: Dr. Elisabeth Beyer Nolen, runner and physician, "Menopause and Exercise," unpublished AMAA Boston Marathon Sports Medicine Symposium talk.

CHAPTER 16 Young at Heart

248 quarter of children engage in physical activity: U.S. Centers for Disease Control and Prevention statistics.

249 are ineligible to serve: Thomas Spoehr and Bridget Handy, "The Looming National Security Crisis: Young Americans Unable to Serve in the Military," Heritage Foundation *Backgrounder,* no. 3282, February 13, 2018.

249 The JFK 50 Mile was born: For historical information and links on the JFK 50 Mile, see "Take the JFK/Freedom's Run challenge . . ." on the Natural Running Center website, naturalrunningcenter.com.

250 cascades of growth factors: C. W. Cotman, N. C. Berchtold, and L. A. Christie, "Exercise Builds Brain Health: Key Roles of Growth Factor Cascades and Inflammation," *Trends in Neuroscience* 30 (2007): 464–72.

252 *zero* days missed: See Mick Grant, *The Youth and Teen Running Encyclopedia: A Complete Guide for Middle and Long Distance Runners Ages 6 to 18.* Grant is an exercise physiologist for the U.S. Air Force and a lifelong coach for youth.

CHAPTER 17 Healthy at Any Age

259 *Once, when I was a young physician*: Gretchen Reynolds, "See How Exercise Keeps Us Young," *New York Times,* January 7, 2015.

260 physical activity has a protective effect: A. Z. Burzynska et al., "Physical Ac-

tivity Is Linked to Greater Moment-to-Moment Variability in Spontaneous Brain Activity in Older Adults," *PLoS ONE* 10, no. 8 (2015).

260 A Stanford study found: F. S. Facchini et al., "Insulin Resistance as a Predictor of Age-Related Diseases," *Journal of Clinical Endocrinology and Metabolism* 86, no. 8 (2001): 3574–78. "The fact that an age-related clinical event developed in approximately 1 out of 3 healthy individuals in the upper tertile of insulin resistance at baseline, followed for an average of 6 years, whereas no clinical events were observed in the most insulin-sensitive tertile, should serve as a strong stimulus to further efforts to define the role of insulin resistance in the genesis of age-related diseases."

260 Dr. Dale Bredesen and colleagues: Dale E. Bredesen et al., "Reversal of Cognitive Decline in Alzheimer's Disease," *Aging* 8, no. 6 (June 2016). I also recommend dementia specialist Bredesen's recent book *The End of Alzheimer's*, which describes thirty years of research and clinical work on the factors that lead to this condition.

261–62 Dallas Bedrest and Training Study: D. K. McGuire et al., "A 30-year Follow-up of the Dallas Bedrest and Training Study: II. Effect of Age on Cardiovascular Adaptation to Exercise Training," *Circulation* 104, no. 12 (2001): 1358–66.

264 MRIs below: Vonda Wright, "Chronic Exercise Preserves Lean Muscle Mass in Masters Athletes." *The Physician and Sports Medicine* 39(3)2011:172–3.

264 two weeks of limitations on walking: Rikke Krogh-Madsen et al., "A 2-Week Reduction of Ambulatory Activity Attenuates Peripheral Insulin Sensitivity," *Journal of Applied Physiology* 108 (2010): 1034–40.

268 running and other impact sports: D. J. Hunter and F. Eckstein, "Exercise and Osteoarthritis," *Journal of Anatomy* 214 (2009): 197–207.

268 multiple marathons annually: Paul T. Williams, "Effects of Running and Walking on Osteoarthritis and Hip Replacement Risk," *Medicine and Science in Sports and Exercise* 45, no. 7 (2013): 1292–97.

268 "The list of diseases that exercise": Chi-Pang Wen et al., "Minimal Amount of Exercise to Prolong Life: To Walk, to Run, or Just Mix It Up?," *Journal of the American College of Cardiology* 64, no. 5 (2014).

268 addition of three years to life expectancy: D. Lee et al., "Leisure-Time Running Reduces All-Cause and Cardiovascular Mortality Risk," *Journal of the American College of Cardiology* 64 (2014): 472–81. See also C. P. Wen et al., "Minimum Amount of Physical Activity for Reduced Mortality and Extended Life Expectancy: A Prospective Cohort Study," *Lancet* 378 (2011): 1244–53.

270 Healthy, long telomeres: Elizabeth Fernandez, "Lifestyle Changes May Lengthen Telomeres, a Measure of Cell Aging," *UCSF News Center*, San Francisco, September 16, 2013. See also teloyears.com. (If you take the test and your "teloyears" are higher than your actual age, don't worry: following the simple health tips in this book will help change that.)

CHAPTER 18 The Nature Cure

271 *In many modern societies*: Helen Santiago Fink, "Human-Nature for Climate Action: Nature-Based Solutions for Urban Sustainability," *Sustainability* 8, no. 3 (2016): 254.

272 A study by Frances Kuo: Frances E. Kuo and Andrea Faber Taylor, "A Po-

tential Natural Treatment for Attention-Deficit/Hyperactivity Disorder: Evidence from a National Study," *American Journal of Public Health* 94, no. 9 (2004).

273 Experiments performed by Marc Berman: Marc G. Berman, John Jonides, and Stephen Kaplan, "The Cognitive Benefits of Interacting with Nature," *Psychological Science* 19, no. 12 (2008): 1207–12.

273 Ruth Ann Atchley and colleagues: R. A. Atchley, D. L. Strayer, and P. Atchley, "Creativity in the Wild: Improving Creative Reasoning Through Immersion in Natural Settings," *PLoS ONE* 7, no. 12 (2012).

273 ninety-minute walk through a natural environment: Gregory N. Bratman et al., "Nature Experience Reduces Rumination and Subgenual Prefrontal Cortex Activation," *Proceedings of the National Academy of Sciences USA* 112, no. 28 (2015): 8567–72.

274 dedicated to improving public health: Visit the Nature Prescriptions site (natureprescriptions.org), and its *Discover the Forest* site (discovertheforest .org), which includes a park finder by zip code. For kids, especially, the National Environmental Education Foundation (neefusa.org) and the Children & Nature Network (childrenandnature.org), started by Richard Louv, offer more information about getting outside.

274 reconnected to the natural world: A rich medical literature exists on the beneficial effects of nature, outdoor activity, play, and access to parks on children's health, communication skills, creativity, cooperation, civility, harmony, and cognitive performance. For instance, see K. Van Der Horst et al., "A Brief Review on Correlates of Physical Activity and Sedentariness in Youth," *Medicine and Science in Sports and Exercise* 39, no. 8 (2007): 1241–50.

275 a coalition of health providers: Visit the National ParkRx Initiative site (parkrx.org), and Park Rx America (parkrxamerica.org).

275 Jennifer Wolch and colleagues: Jennifer Wolch et al., "Childhood Obesity and Proximity to Urban Parks and Recreational Resources: A Longitudinal Cohort Study," *Health & Place* 17, no. 1 (2011): 207–14.

CHAPTER 19 Running in Place

282 *a culture of physical activity*: Chi-Pang Wen et al., "Minimal Amount of Exercise to Prolong Life: To Walk, to Run, or Just Mix It Up?," *Journal of the American College of Cardiology* 64, no. 5 (2014). "[I]nactivity can lead to a 25% increase in heart disease and a 45% increase in cardiovascular disease mortality, not to mention a 10% increase in the incidence of cancer, diabetes, and untold depression."

284 "Determinants of Health": See the World Health Organization's Health Impact Assessment, www.who.int/hia/evidence/doh/en/.

284 The corollary is also true: J. T. Cacioppo and S. Cacioppo, "Social Relationships and Health: The Toxic Effects of Perceived Social Isolation," *Social and Personality Psychology Compass* 8, no. 2 (2014): 58–72.

286 *one-third* the amount spent on food: See "How Much Does the U.S. Spend on Health and How Has It Changed?," Henry J. Kaiser Family Foundation, May 1, 2012, www.kff.org/report-section/health-care-costs-a-primer-2012 -report/. See also Culinary Institute of America and Harvard T. H. Chan School of Public Health, www.menusofchange.org/principles-resources/

issue-briefs/healthy-food-vs-healthcare-spending-and-trends-in-medical
-culinary-educati.

286   *more than double* what they spent on food: Ricardo Alonso-Zaldivar, "$10,345
       per Person: U.S. Health Care Spending Reaches New Peak," Associated Press,
       July 13, 2016.

Index

hydration, 72, 177
hyperglycemia, 145
hyponatremia, 190
hysteresis, 64

Iditarod Trail, 276
iliotibial band syndrome (ITBS), 218
impact moderating behavior (IMB),
    215
Independent Running Retail
    Association, 288
inflammation, 171–73
    diet and, 138, 144–45, 147, 172
    NSAIDs for, 172, 215, 222, 223,
    229
injuries, xiv, 77–78, 107, 213–15,
    282
    cascades of, 214
    causes and symptoms of, 219
    common, 218–21
    and level of exertion, 217
    overstriding and, 83–84
    rest for, 224–25
    without pain, 214
    See also specific injuries
injury prevention, viii, xiv, 213–29
    drills for, 228–29
    impact moderating behavior, 215
    mobility work, 217
    prehab, 216–17
    video recording your movement, 228
instability, 119–20
insulin, 8, 144–45, 148, 149, 151,
    164, 165, 176, 188
    resistance, 141–49, 151, 154, 161,
    163, 164, 176, 206, 236–37, 245,
    260, 261
    sensitivity, 141, 164
Ioannidis, John P. A., 159
intervals, 11, 322
intestinal microbiome, 205–6, 250
Inuit, 8
iron, 238, 245
Ironman races, 173, 186
isolation training, 117
IT band syndrome, 65, 241

Jefferson Medical Center, 157, 161
JFK 50 Mile, 249

jogging:
    family, 283
    See also slow jogging
joints, 77, 213, 214
Jordan, Michael, 23
*Journal of the American College of
    Cardiology,* 268
*Journal of the American Medical
    Association,* 142
jumping jacks, 258
jump ropes, 95, 256, 258

kale and walnut pesto, 170
Kalenjin, 8
Karvonen formula, 111
Katovsky, Bill, 202
Kawauchi, Yuki, 200
Keflezighi, Meb, 122–23, 185
Kennedy, John F., 160, 217, 247, 249,
    280, 289
Kennedy, Robert F., 249
Kenyans:
    runners, xi, 8, 19, 164
    women who carry loads on their
    heads, 33
Kerrigan, Casey, x
ketogenic diet, 177
ketone bodies, 102
Keys, Ancel, 152, 153
King, Martin Luther, Jr., 31
Kipchoge, Eliud, 194
knee, 92, 214, 241
    pain in, 92
    valgus, 220–21, 241, 245
kneeling, 21, 131
Kotelko, Olga, 67
Kowalchik, Claire, 233
Krebs cycle, 100
Kuhn, Hans-George, 250
Kulund, Daniel, x
Kuo, Frances, 272

laboratory tests, 156–57
lactate threshold (anaerobic threshold),
    103, 104–6, 111
Lawrence Berkeley National
    Laboratory, 268
LDL (low-density lipoprotein),
    153–54, 266

triglycerides, 20, 99, 100, 141
TrueForm Runner, 91–92, 229
Two Rivers Treads store, vii, xi, 55, 67, 91, 220, 288–89
Tulu, Derartu, 235
Tunis, John, 234
Turkish Getup, 137

University of Colorado, 241
University of Gothenburg, 250
University of Illinois, 260
University of Michigan, 273
USDA, 287

van Lingen, Lawrence, 69, 70
vegetarian or vegan diets, 239
ventilatory threshold (VT) or aerobic threshold (AeT), 103, 105
Vernikos, Joan, 20, 21
vestibular system, 5–6
vitamins:
    B_{12}, 246
    D, 238, 245
    K and K_2, 245
VO_2 max, 105–6, 112–13, 262, 264

walking, 8, 31–42, 119, 203, 268
    accessories for, 39–40
    barefoot, 55, 223
    drills for, 41–42
    mixing running with, 40
    shoes for, 37–39
walnut and kale pesto, 170
water, drinking, 72, 177, 199
    dehydration and, 198
    too much, 190, 197, 198
water, soaking in, 72–73, 183
web resources, 291
weight, 138, 147, 150, 162, 165
    waist size and, 142, 147, 154, 164
    See also obesity
weight loss, 164–66, 206
    diets for, 158–59
weightlessness, 20–21
Weight Watchers, 158–59
Weinstock, David, 115

Welch, Priscilla, 233
Wen, Chi-Pang, 282
West Virginia, xv, 166–67, 208, 250, 284, 285
    Eastern Area Health Education Center in, 251
    Freedom's Run in. See Freedom's Run
    Two Rivers Treads store in, vii, xi, 55, 67, 91, 220, 288–89
West Virginia University (WVU), vii, xvi, 24, 167, 287
What Makes Olga Run? (Grierson), 67
Williams, Paul, 268
windshield wiper progression, 133
Winfrey, Oprah, 159, 236
Wolch, Jennifer, 275
women, 233–46
    adolescence and, 239–41, 255
    bone density in, 237–38
    C-sections in, 241
    drills for, 245–46
    hormones and, 236–39, 241–42
    in marathons, 235–36
    medical issues and, 236–39
    menopause in, 241–42
    menstrual dysregulation in, 238
    nutrition and, 236–39, 245–46
    nutritional imbalance or insufficiency in, 237
    osteoporosis and, 233
    performance gap between men and, 236
    pregnancy and, 233, 237, 241, 245
    RED-S and, 237–38, 240, 242
    stress and, 242–43
    Ubuntu concept and, 235
Women's Health Initiative, 241–42
World Health Organization, 284

Yessis, Michael, x
yoga ball, 26

zero gravity, 20–21
Zero Runner, 229
zoning in, 211
zoning out, 211

ILLUSTRATION CREDITS

A NOTE ON THE TYPE

This book was set in Adobe Garamond. Designed for the Adobe Corporation by Robert Slimbach, the fonts are based on types first cut by Claude Garamond (c. 1480–1561). Garamond was a pupil of Geoffroy Tory and is believed to have followed the Venetian models, although he introduced a number of important differences, and it is to him that we owe the letter we now know as "old style." He gave to his letters a certain elegance and feeling of movement that won their creator an immediate reputation and the patronage of Francis I of France.

Composed by North Market Street Graphics
Lancaster, Pennsylvania

Printed and bound by Berryville Graphics
Berryville, Virginia

Designed by Maggie Hinders